Conquering Chronic Pain after Injury

Conquering Chronic Pain after Injury

An Integrative Approach to Treating Post-Traumatic Pain

WILLIAM H. SIMON, M.D.,
GEORGE E. EHRLICH, M.D.,
and
ARNOLD SADWIN, M.D.

AVERY
a member of Penguin Putnam Inc.
New York

Every effort has been made to ensure that the information contained in this book is complete and accurate. However, neither the publisher nor the authors are engaged in rendering professional advice or services to the individual reader. The ideas, procedures, and suggestions contained in this book are not intended as a substitute for consulting with your physician. All matters regarding health require medical supervision. Neither the authors nor the publisher shall be liable or responsible for any loss, injury, or damage allegedly arising from any information or suggestion in this book. The opinions expressed in this book represent the personal views of the authors and not of the publisher.

While the authors have made every effort to provide accurate telephone numbers and Internet addresses at the time of publication, neither the publisher nor the authors assume any responsibility for errors or for changes that occur after publication.

Most Avery books are available at special quantity discounts for bulk purchase for sales promotions, premiums, fund-raising, and educational needs. Special books or book excerpts also can be created to fit specific needs. For details, write Putnam Special Markets, 375 Hudson Street, New York, NY 10014.

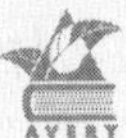

a member of
Penguin Putnam Inc.
375 Hudson Street
New York, NY 10014
www.penguinputnam.com

Library of Congress Cataloging-in-Publication Data

Conquering chronic pain after injury : an integrative approach to treating post-traumatic pain / William H. Simon, George E. Ehrlich, and Arnold Sadwin [editors].
p. cm.
ISBN 1-58333-140-9
1. Alternative medicine. 2. Chronic pain—Treatment. 3. Pain—Alternative treatment. 4. Post-traumatic stress disorder—Treatment. I. Simon, William H. (William Herson), date. II. Ehrlich, George E. III. Sadwin, Arnold.
R733.O937 2002 2002023230
616'.0472—dc21

Printed in the United States of America

1 3 5 7 9 10 8 6 4 2

Book design by Tanya Maiboroda

CONTENTS

To my modern muse, Michele

—WHS

To Gail, Steven and Debbie, Rebecca and David, and Charles

—GEE

To Sue, Donna, Stuart, Valerie, Lori, Paul, Michael, Allison, Kelly, and Moya

—AS

ACKNOWLEDGMENTS

The authors wish to acknowledge the invaluable assistance of Nancy Steele, our medical editor; Dara Stewart, our editor at Avery; and Blanche Schlessinger, our superb literary agent.

Dr. Simon would like to acknowledge the efforts of his hardworking staff: Estelle, Debbie B., Debbie G., Pat, and Ruth.

Dr. Sadwin would like to acknowledge the help of Rhona Paul-Cohen, an expert in cognitive remediation, John Gordon, Ph.D., David Masseri, Ph.D., Kathy Lawler, Psy.D., and Joely Esposito, Psy.D., neuropsychologists, for their help; Pamela Schmid for her transcription work; Erick Snyder for his graphics help; Donna Sadwin and Lorraine Mance for their help in assembling the manuscript; and his wife, Sue Matney-Sadwin, and his daughter, Lori O'Leary, for their editing help.

FOREWORD

BY DR. BOB ARNOT,
MEDICAL CORRESPONDENT NBC/MSNBC

Here's a first-ever comprehensive approach to a problem not previously focused upon: the painful and emotionally disturbing aftermath of pain after an injury. The lives of millions of Americans, their friends, and their loved ones are adversely affected by this unrelenting and difficult-to-treat pain.

Here you'll find the answers to frequently asked questions about Post-traumatic Pain Syndrome:

1. What causes it?
2. How do you explain the disease states associated with it?
3. How does a sufferer get better?
4. What role does Alternative or Complementary Medicine play?
5. How can yoga, diet, herbal medicine, or chiropractic treatment help?

The authors provide help and encouragement to help you overcome pain in order to win back your life.

We all know people who have suffered for years after a serious auto accident or work-related injury. An orthopedic surgeon (Dr. Simon), a rheumatologist (Dr. Ehrlich), and a neuropsychiatrist (Dr. Sadwin) have written an especially useful book that removes the mystery of chronic pain after injury—and approaches the solutions from physical, emotional, and metaphysical vantage points.

These skilled academic physicians draw from experts who would not ordinarily combine their skills into a single endeavor. This book is unique because it willingly accepts methodologies and techniques from diverse sources in order to produce the most holistic approach to the solution of chronic post-traumatic pain thus far available to the sufferer.

The authors also remove the myths and prejudices surrounding the emotional and psychological effects of one of the unspoken causes of suffering for millions of patients and their families in America today.

This book is designed so that those sufferers from chronic post-traumatic pain can reach their goal of obtaining relief. The road to relief, however, is not a one-way street. Doctors Simon, Ehrlich, and Sadwin encourage the reader, you, to become an active participant in your own recovery.

Ultimately, drawing on ancient mythology, the authors display a firm belief in the curative powers of Hope. As an informed patient with an optimistic outlook, you can help maximize your own cure. Case histories and even a doctor's own story of recovery help dramatize the human struggle to regain one's health and happiness, and once more become an active participant in work, family, and community life.

Conquering Chronic Pain after Injury is a continuing reference source for the persons and their families who are struggling to overcome post-traumatic pain.

If you wish to know why you still hurt, even after treatment for a painful injury is over; if you have a desire to know whether the reasons for your continued pain have been adequately explained; if you have been made to feel as if you were just a chronic complainer, when you know there is actually something painfully wrong with you; if you wish to know if all available methods of help have been offered to you: then this is the book for you!

INTRODUCTION

According to ancient Greek myth, Pandora was a beautiful woman who was given to one of the Titans as a gift of the gods. Along with Pandora, the gods sent a sealed box that was to be kept closed at all costs. When Pandora's curiosity got the best of her, she opened the box, and out flew pain, disease, and all the other evils of the world. By the time Pandora closed the lid, all that remained inside the box was hope. It is said that ever since, humans have cherished hope as a powerful weapon to conquer the pain of life.

The message of this book is hope—hope for those 14 million Americans annually who suffer traumatic injuries and endure persistent pain despite long-term medical care, and hope for their families who suffer along with them.

In this book, the authors offer not only hope but also the expectation of a good outcome. Although you may not be able to find quick relief from your pain, and perhaps not even a cure, you'll discover that you can improve your condition by taking charge of your care, by exploring a wide choice of treatments, and by making certain lifestyle adjustments.

The principal authors of this book are orthopedic surgeon William

H. Simon, M.D., rheumatologist George E. Ehrlich, M.D., and neuropsychiatrist Arnold Sadwin, M.D. Each of these physicians has more than three decades of experience in treating thousands of patients who have post-traumatic pain. In this book, these three experts, together with other practitioners whose specialties include both traditional and alternative medicine, offer advice to help answer the two questions most often asked by those who suffer from post-traumatic pain: "Why do I still hurt?" and "What can I do about it?"

Many patients whose injuries appear to have been adequately cared for continue to suffer pain even after their fractures and lacerations have healed, after their head injuries and disc herniations have been treated, and after their muscles, ligaments, and tendons have been rehabilitated. Often their physicians tell them, "There is nothing more that I can do for you" or "You'll just have to live with it" or, worst of all, "It's all in your head."

To some extent, all of these statements may be true, but that doesn't help the patient to feel better. This book provides a holistic approach to solving this predicament: We will consider both physical and mental explanations for persistent post-traumatic pain, fatigue, and weakness.

It is a fact that all pain is in our heads. Without the brain to interpret certain signals from the body and from the brain itself, we would feel no pain. But even though our brains allow us to feel pain, we also can use our brains to defend us against pain and to help us cope with the powerful stimuli that cause pain.

In order to explain how post-traumatic pain syndrome can affect you, we will consider three types of conditions: mind over body; body over mind; and mind over mind.

Mind-over-body conditions occur when external circumstances affect a patient's mental outlook and aggravate, or even provoke, further physical problems such as increased pain or decreased physical ability. Circumstances that can have a profound effect upon mental outlook include the inability to maintain a normal working routine due to injury or the loss of economic and social status due to a serious injury to the family's main breadwinner.

Body-over-mind conditions are the opposite of mind-over-body conditions. Body (or somatic) dysfunction (such as scarring or nerve irritation) can produce debilitating mental attitudes such as depression and fatigue.

Mind-over-mind conditions are rare, but they too are discussed in this book. These include malingering and conversion. *Malingering* is a voluntary, intentional response in which an accident victim pretends to be more seriously hurt than he or she really is, for an external incentive. The second response, *conversion,* is an involuntary, subconscious one in which a person truly believes that he or she is physically impaired, but the physical findings don't confirm this.

USING THIS BOOK

In order to explore these three conditions, we have divided this book into two parts. Part One: Why Do I Still Hurt? will help you to begin the process of overcoming the "lonesome syndrome" of post-traumatic pain.

Understanding the causes of your pain—causes not simply due to contusions, sprains, strains, fractures, dislocations, disc herniations, or nerve injuries—will allow you to begin the process of coping with your physical and emotional conditions. In this part, we explore the difficulties of diagnosing and treating post-traumatic conditions that lead to persistent pain. Both the physician and the patient share responsibility for coming to the right conclusions, and the role that the patient can play in contributing to the proper diagnosis and treatment is emphasized. The diagnosis and treatment of unusual or rare diseases as they relate to post-traumatic pain also are explained, to the extent that they are currently understood.

Of course, not every cause of persistent pain can be dealt with in a book of this size. However, in Part One, we will explore the most common causes of persistent pain, in chapters written by physicians who are experts in studying and treating the elements of post-traumatic pain syndrome—post-traumatic stress syndrome, post-concussion syndrome, hidden-disc syndrome, referred-pain syndrome, fibromyalgia, chronic fatigue and chronic pain syndrome, and reflex sympathetic dystrophy. Within this part, you should find useful information about your own post-traumatic pain syndrome.

In Part Two: What Can I Do About It? you'll find information that will give you hope, help you to recondition your mind and body, and enable you to regain a life of activity and usefulness. This section emphasizes choices of treatment for post-traumatic pain, both traditional and alternative. These treatments include drug therapy, psychotherapy, cognitive therapy, chiropractic care, nutritional therapy, yoga, bodywork techniques such as t'ai chi and Rolfing, biofeedback, acupuncture, and trigger-release therapy. In each chapter, an expert in one of these fields describes successful methods in treating some or all of the conditions explored in Part One.

Now let us return to the premise of this book—hope. Consider the tale of the ancient Greek archer Philoctetes, as dramatized by the playwright Sophocles. Philoctetes, the supreme Greek archer in the Trojan War, was bitten on the heel by a snake, and his wound festered. The unbearable pain caused him to cry out in despair. His fellow warriors felt that he was a detriment to the battle, and they exiled him to the island of Lemnos. There, he lived alone in pain and without hope.

On the battlefield, things were not going well for the Greeks. Odysseus, one of the leaders of the Greeks, went to Lemnos to persuade Philoctetes to return to the battle and fire his magic arrows, despite his disabling wound. Philoctetes, depressed and in constant pain, declined to follow Odysseus. Then Apollo, the Greek god of healing, appeared to Philoctetes and promised that if he would return to the battle, his painful wound would be healed forever.

Filled with hope, Philoctetes rejoined his comrades in battle. He fired his arrows, and the Greeks prevailed. As promised, his debilitating wound healed—a triumph of hope over pain and misery.

The authors of this book trust that, like Philoctetes and Pandora, you will find within these pages the hope you need to triumph in your own battle against pain.

William H. Simon, M.D.

PART

1

WHY DO I STILL HURT?

IF YOU have experienced unrelenting post-traumatic pain, you may be frustrated and angry—angry with your doctor for not being able to cure your pain, angry with your insurance company for not covering your ongoing medical expenses, or angry with the person or people who played a part in your injury. You probably are frustrated that you continue to suffer and are unable to return to your pre-accident level of activity.

The first part of this book will attempt to calm some of your anger and frustration by providing logical, scientifically based evidence to explain the persistence of your pain. Knowledge is a powerful tool. In this case, knowing the reasons for your pain can set you on the right path toward understanding your condition and inspire you to adopt behaviors and actions that will give you relief. You'll learn how you can begin to do this in Part Two: What Can I Do About It?

Should you be angry with your doctors for their failure to cure you? Or should you be angry with yourself for not getting better? Well, maybe both, or maybe neither. Let us explore both situations.

YOUR DOCTOR'S ROLE

Assuming that your doctor has done the very best to help heal your injuries—fractures, dislocations, bruises, sprains, strains, lacerations, contusions, and disc herniations—what more do you expect from your physician?

First of all, you expect your doctor to spend some time with you and to listen to you. That sounds simple, but in this era of managed care, the pressure on physicians to treat as many patients as they can each day puts tight limits on the amount of time they have to spend with each patient. This often makes it difficult to take a detailed history from you concerning your persistent pains and physical disabilities. This is particularly true after your initial evaluation, which establishes your injuries and sets out a program to treat them.

According to Zelda Di Blasi, M.D., of the University of York in the United Kingdom, doctors who showed empathy and who acknowledged their patients' fears and anxieties were more effective than doctors who kept their patients at emotional arm's length. Dr. Di Blasi says that a sense of partnership and trust should be nurtured and thought of as part of the health-care package. But, she says, the current system discourages continuity of care and does not allow enough time for a healing interaction.

Often, doctors are more concerned with *objective findings*—symptoms that can be seen or felt or measured—than they are with *subjective complaints,* such as pain, numbness, fatigue, or weakness, which can sound more like complaints than true medical symptoms.

Some physicians tend to focus on their fields of expertise—the spine, bones, joints, hands, or nerves—rather than consider the patient as a total person with a holistic approach. After all, your doctor may have no idea how you functioned before your injury, how hard you worked, or how much you enjoyed the sports activities in which you are no longer capable of participating. Also, doctors who are experts in one area of the body may skip over or ignore symptoms that are not related to their specialty, or they may not consider a diagnosis that has its origin in other areas of specialty. For example, an orthopedic surgeon may not diagnose a condition that a neurologist normally treats. Finally, some doctors are such super-specialists that once they have completed their "work" on your fracture or your head injury, they feel that they really have done all they can for you.

YOUR ROLE

What can you do as a patient to help yourself? What is your responsibility to yourself and to your doctor in treating your post-traumatic pain?

First, ask yourself, "What is my problem today?" Write out your symptoms and make your answer clear, concise, and complete. Second, don't have a hidden agenda. Tell your physician the whole story. Don't conveniently "forget" the accident that required a year's treatment before your last injury. Concentrate on the medical problem with your doctor, not the employment problem, the insurance problem, or the legal problem.

Third, don't test your doctor. Don't play the game "You're the doctor—you figure out what's wrong with me!" This is a hostile attitude and, in many cases, will provoke a hostile reaction from your doctor. That is no way to start a successful doctor-patient relationship. Be cooperative: Help your doctor make the proper diagnosis. Don't exaggerate your symptoms, but don't dismiss symptoms that might be clues to the cause of your pain—odd feelings, weakness, or a sense of fatigue.

Finally, don't expect an instant cure. As the saying goes, "Great expectations, great disappointments." When you work with your doctors, not against them, you have the best chance of getting the best results.

FINDING THE CAUSE OF PAIN

The chapters in this part concentrate on problems that are difficult to diagnose and that cause persistent post-traumatic pain—pain that just won't go away. If the reason for the pain were simple, either physical or mental, you wouldn't need this book. Therefore, the experts in the chapters that follow concentrate on some difficult, if not rare, reasons for pain. You may find the answer to why you still hurt in one of these chapters, and in all of them you will find important information about the origins of post-traumatic pain.

Chapter 1: Understanding Post-Traumatic Pain provides a basic introduction to the subject. In this chapter, Dr. Simon translates the language of post-traumatic pain and provides signposts to help you locate yourself among those who suffer from this condition.

In Chapter 2: Hidden-Disc and Referred-Pain Syndromes, Dr. Simon focuses on two medical conditions that are often difficult for patients (and even for some physicians) to accept as causes of prolonged post-traumatic pain. The first of these is an injury to the spine that can't be detected by the most sophisticated methods known to modern medicine. The second of these conditions is an injury to one part of the body that causes pain in a different part of the body that is perfectly healthy.

In Chapter 3: Fibromyalgia, Chronic Pain, and Fatigue, Dr. Ehrlich explores several post-traumatic conditions that have no known physical cause and no known cure. These conditions are distinguished by subjective symptoms such as tenderness in multiple "trigger points" throughout the body, feelings of weakness and fatigue, and insomnia. Anyone who has been diagnosed as having chronic pain or fatigue will be most interested in Dr. Ehrlich's explanations and discussion.

Chapter 4: Hidden Concussions, by Dr. Sadwin, provides information about the physical and emotional problems that can be caused by a head injury—even when the patient is unaware that a head injury has occurred. In this chapter, you'll find forty symptoms that point to a head injury. Personality changes can be caused by a head injury, so if someone tells you that you are not your old self since your injury, be sure to read this chapter carefully.

In Chapter 5: Complex Regional Pain Syndrome (CRPS) or Reflex Sympathetic Dystrophy (RSD), Sanjay Gupta, M.D., a pain specialist, presents the most current findings and explanations for a condition that is as painful as it is difficult to understand. Reflex sympathetic dystrophy, or RSD, is thought by some investigators to represent a dysfunction of the autonomic nervous system of the body, brought about by trauma. You may find the explanation for your unusual post-traumatic condition in this informative chapter.

Chapter 6: Mind/Body, Body/Mind, Mind/Brain, and Post-Traumatic Stress Disorder (PTSD) by Joseph C. Napoli, M.D., a psychiatrist and an expert on post-traumatic stress, explains how the mind and the body can interact to produce chronic pain after an injury. If you read this chapter carefully, somewhere in it you may find a reference to what is happening to you or to someone in your family.

In this book, you'll also find a first-person account by family physician Elizabeth Michel, M.D., who tells how her life dramatically changed after she was struck by a car. The story of how she conquered her pain and learned to heal will inform and inspire you. The first part of her story, "A Doctor's Own Story of Trauma," follows. You'll find the second part, "A Doctor's Own Story of Healing," as part of the introduction to Part Two.

William H. Simon, M.D.

A DOCTOR'S OWN STORY OF TRAUMA

ELIZABETH MICHEL, M.D.

On November 12, 1980, my life cracked into two eras. For many years thereafter, I called these eras "Before the Accident" and "After the Accident." In my mind, I saw them as the two halves of a pot that had cracked from top to bottom. The pot was still upright; someone looking at it from a distance would see a whole pot. But it could not do the work of a pot; its usefulness had been destroyed by the jagged space of a dark, ugly crack.

To this day, I cannot remember my accident, but I have been told what happened. It was a beautiful day, and I was hoping to run five miles before it ended. But when I came home from my morning clinic, I had to wait for an appointment with my piano tuner. He arrived late, and by the time he finished his work, there was not enough time for my usual five-mile run. My husband would need my help when he came home with two hungry children after a long day at his own clinic. But we were almost out of milk, so I decided to run just two miles and pick up the milk on my way home. I folded a dollar bill, slipped it into the tiny inner pocket of my running shorts, and ran out our gate feeling exhilarated by my repaired piano, the California sunshine, and the bodily pleasure of running.

Filled with joyful expectation, I ran down the hill near my house and turned toward the beach. The next thing I remember is waking up and seeing my friend Steve from my residency program standing over me in surgical scrubs. I was frightened and very confused. Steve calmed me and explained what had happened, but it was some time before I comprehended. I had been hit by a car, and both of my legs were broken.

My legs, both encased in casts, hurt terribly, and I could not move. My arms were taped to boards; cold fluid was running into both of my arms through IV tubes. An oxygen tube ran into my nose, and a catheter was running from my bladder. My clothes had been cut off my body, and I was naked and shivering under a thin sheet.

Soon a police officer came to my side and filled me in on the details of the accident. I had been waiting by a pedestrian crosswalk when the driver of a van stopped to let me cross. As I started to cross, I couldn't see the smaller car on the other side of the van. It barreled through the crosswalk at full speed—illegally—and hit me. The impact threw me seventy to ninety feet into the air. Someone called 911 from the little Mexican restaurant on the other side of the street.

The ambulance arrived quickly, and the hospital was close. Otherwise, I might have bled to death. In fact, before sophisticated trauma-response systems came into being in the 1970s, most victims of serious accidents did die. Thus I became a survivor at a time when little was known about the long-term challenges such survivors would face.

Planning a Full Recovery

Once I regained consciousness and realized that I had narrowly escaped being killed, I was filled with an expansive optimism I had never felt before. Perhaps I was feeling the effect of the large dose of morphine I had been given; more likely, massive psychological denial had set in. I "knew" that I was going to recover completely. I did have some medical knowledge that would have contradicted my optimism, but I conveniently forgot it.

When the orthopedist arrived, he showed me my X-rays and explained my injuries. The car had directly struck my left lower leg. It was a very bad break: The bone there—the tibia—was in many pieces, and a deep wound through the skin and muscle left the bone vulnerable to infection. One of the fracture lines extended into the knee joint. Surgery was needed to clean the wound, align the pieces of bone, and stabilize them by inserting orthopedic "pins" (a euphemism—they were the size of large nails) through my bones above and below the fracture. My right tibia had sustained a simpler fracture and did not require surgery. I also had a concussion, bruised kidneys, and deep abrasions along the right side of my body where I had hit the pavement after my long flight through the air.

Steve called my husband, Arnie, who had just arrived home with the children. Ten minutes later, Arnie walked into the emergency room with one little boy on each arm. Arnie asked the police officer if the accident had been my fault. The officer replied, "No," then added, "but she could have been more careful." In general, I had been a careful person; the sum total of my prior treatment for injuries had been five stitches at the tip of a finger that had come too close to a kitchen knife. Still, it would be many years before I would stop feeling that this accident, in which someone else had broken a law, was my fault.

I don't remember much else from this time. I was in pain, my thinking was clouded, and I was very weak. But I continued to feel optimistic about recovering and going back to running. I would work hard at my rehabilitation. My determination would see me through. My mind went to extremes to deny the seriousness of my injuries. When the director of my clinic called me the day after the accident, I told him that I would be back at work as soon as I was allowed up on crutches! I did not think about how I would get around the clinic with a cast on each leg.

Two days after the accident, I was transferred to the hospital at which Arnie practiced as an internist. There, a physical therapist taught me how to move my torso between the bed and a wheelchair while someone lifted my legs. Arnie came up to see me whenever he could take a break from his work.

My casts were so heavy that I could not even turn myself in bed, so someone would have to take care of me when I went home. The thought of a stranger helping me in the bathroom distressed me greatly, but my sister, Cynthia, a nurse, wanted to care for me, and she was able to arrange to take a month's leave from her job.

I spent nine days in the hospital. Before my discharge, a social worker recommended to my orthopedist that a visiting nurse see me at home at least once to assess my situation. The orthopedist refused to order the visit because my sister was a nurse. Later, I realized that he had denied me badly needed practical and emotional support from someone with expertise. Cynthia cared lovingly for me, but she was a labor and delivery nurse who had little experience with the problems I was facing.

A Sense of Loss

For years after the accident, I believed that I could cure my pain and disability by working stubbornly at rehabilitating myself, and the orthopedist and physical therapist who treated me during the early years did not suggest otherwise. As a result, I suffered unnecessary pain and anguish, in part because I fought too hard against letting go of what I could not do, and in part because post-accident problems were poorly understood at that time and no one was trained to help me let go.

Like most people, I have found it hard to let go of things that seem important. Sometimes, I have felt that nothing would ever replace what was being wrenched from me. I have felt that I had to have *this* person, or *that* means of expressing my identity, in my life. I have felt empty without this or that, and I have felt shamed in the eyes of others by my emptiness. I have felt alone, abandoned, and unloved.

My lengthy recuperation has taught me to take a more long-term view of loss. In the immediate aftermath of the accident, only one person I knew, an older colleague, understood what endless patience I would need. "You will keep getting better for years and years," he said. This friend's life was an example of what "getting better" has come to mean to me. No longer able to practice medicine after a distinguished career, he kept himself connected, through new interests, to other people and to his own passion for life.

I was still young, but eventually I, too, was forced to accept that I could no longer take care of patients. I was in pain and depressed; the pace at the clinic was too hard for me, and my children needed every bit of my now-diminished energy. But the pain of letting go of my hard-won professional identity was as excruciating as the exhaustion of clinging to it. My inner conflict lasted for years and conjured the stern faces of physicians scolding, "What? You took up a place at medical school and now you're not going to practice?" But slowly, my training as a physician was integrated into other work that came looking for me, and the things I lost were restored to me in deeply satisfying, though unexpected, forms.

As a young physician, I had had two patients who told me that surviving a life-threatening event had drastically—and positively—shifted their perspectives on the purpose of their lives. I was struck by their words, and I believed them. But I remember these two patients precisely because they puzzled me: Their experiences were beyond my understanding. Then I was forced to experience trauma myself. I didn't complete the shift in perspective that these patients told me about until much later in my recovery, when I found comfort in a psychologist's empathic words: "You are not the same person you were before the accident." Someone finally understood the crack in my world!

After the accident, I felt set apart from "healthy" others by my limitations, and I found that those who had not suffered severe trauma were limited in their ability to grasp what I had been through. I have felt envy and anger toward those others. I also have felt ashamed to discover these feelings within myself. But each time I have accepted these feelings as my own, I have taken giant steps toward healing. Beneath my envy and anger was always grief for what I had lost, and from my grief arose acceptance, and even tenderness, for those others as well as for me.

Healing from serious trauma is difficult in part because an accident is almost never a patient's first deep wound. In the wake of trauma, one's earlier wounds also may need treatment. Different wounds call out for different kinds of healers. Some of my healers have had scientific training; others work from psychological and spiritual perspectives. Some of my healers focused on my physical wounds, the acute fractures that needed repair and the chronically malfunctioning muscles that needed rehabilitation. Some healers helped me with the mental and emotional fragmentation that occurs when head injury and post-traumatic stress disorder (PTSD) complicate trauma. Others helped me to address emotional problems that I had had before my accident, problems that made healing more difficult for me.

A wound, no matter how agonizing it feels when it opens, offers us an opportunity to learn to accept and love ourselves and others as we are: mortal, limited, and less than perfect. The moment that cracked my life into two eras made me feel as helpless as an infant. The accident, like my birth, delivered me, shocked, into a harsher world. Neither delivery left traces in my conscious memory, and I would not have survived either event if others had not cared for me. I have learned to walk twice.

My accident forced me to do the work of repairing wounds I was already carrying when that car hit me. Now I am able to reach out my hand to other trauma survivors and teach them some ways to heal. In the second part of this book, I will show you how I learned to heal my body and how my physical recovery was helped by addressing the emotional and spiritual fractures of my life before the accident.

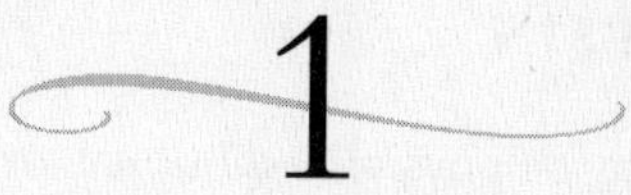

Understanding Post-Traumatic Pain

WILLIAM H. SIMON, M.D.

What is post-traumatic pain syndrome? This term refers to the pain that follows an injury—a fall, an automobile accident, an athletic injury, a work-related injury, or another physical trauma—and the several medical problems that occur at the same time, presenting a group of symptoms both physical and mental.

In this book, we are concerned with a medical problem that has not been "cured" by the usually excellent treatments that are available today. Post-traumatic pain syndrome is pain that persists after all of the standard therapies have been tried, including medication, injections, physical therapy, and surgery; and after none of the usual diagnostic studies give any further information about the cause of the pain.

About three months after an injury, usually all wounds heal, all the black-and-blue marks from contusions and abrasions disappear, and all the physical therapy is complete. But what if the time for sprains and strains to heal has come and gone—and you are still in pain? It's difficult to fix a point in time when healing should be complete, but it's reasonable to venture that if you are still in pain for six months to a year after a traumatic injury, you have post-traumatic pain syndrome, and you need to read this book.

FEELING YOUR PAIN

Post-traumatic pain may be physical, emotional, or both. Emotional pain, such as in post-concussion syndrome, post-traumatic stress syndrome, or chronic pain syndrome, can be just as destructive to your life as persistent pain in your lower back or your feet.

Pain is very individual and can leave a person feeling very lonely. No one else can feel your pain. Each one of us has a different perception of pain. Some of us are stoic; we keep the pain to ourselves, and we don't talk about it to anyone, including our families or even our doctors. This can seemingly be good for those who continue to work and tend to ignore the pain, but sometimes this is a very bad thing because it can lead to severe emotional difficulties and a dysfunctional life. Others complain all the time. We certainly know about their pain because they talk about it incessantly. Most of the time everyone ignores them, and they are no better off than a stoic individual—alone and in pain. You probably recognize yourself somewhere between these two extremes.

SUBJECTIVE AND OBJECTIVE SIGNS OF PAIN

There are two ways to describe findings that point to pain. These are either "subjective" or "objective." A subjective finding is one that only you, the subject, can describe, such as a backache. An objective finding is one that your doctor, or a member of your family, or anyone else who were to examine you, would be able to see, hear, or feel—some physical abnormality about you such as a swelling that might be a symptom of a painful condition. Physicians obtain objective findings by means of physical examinations and diagnostic studies, including X-rays, computerized axial tomography (CAT scans), magnetic resonance imaging (MRIs), electromyograms (EMGs), myelograms, discograms, and electroencephalograms (EEGs).

Too often in post-traumatic pain syndrome, there is an incongruity between the objective findings and the subjective symptoms: Often there are no objective findings to explain the subjective symptoms. This inconsistency makes it that much more difficult to treat post-traumatic pain.

It would be nice if we had a "pain meter" that could register the degree of pain we feel. Unfortunately, all traditional treatment for post-traumatic pain is dependent upon the complete agreement between objective findings and subjective symptoms. Yet in post-traumatic pain syndrome, it's rare that the objective findings entirely explain the subjective symptoms. That's what makes post-traumatic pain so difficult to treat.

DESCRIBING YOUR PAIN

The subjective symptoms of pain can be expressed in many ways. You may feel sharp pain, dull pain, stabbing pain, burning pain, aching pain, radiating pain, or numbness. Many patients feel changes in temperature, either hot or cold, in various parts of their bodies, and others report a sensation similar to running water or ants crawling over their skin.

These sensations are generally referred to as one of the following:

- *hyperesthesia*—an increased sensitivity to stimuli (such as pain felt from stroking, brushing, or lightly touching the skin).
- *dysesthesia*—an abnormal sensation (such as an illusion of hot or cold, ants crawling, or water dripping).
- *paresthesia*—a tingling sensation.
- *hypesthesia*—a decrease in normal sensation.
- *anesthesia*—a loss of sensation.

The sensory nerves in your skin or specialized nerve endings in your muscles, tendons, ligaments, and joints control all of these "pains." These sensations are carried to the spinal cord by the nerves and are almost instantaneously transported to various parts of the brain for interpretation.

Some physicians use drawings or scales to help you describe your pain. The two most common are the Pain Diagram and the Pain Description Scale. The Pain Diagram (see Figure 1.1 on page 16) is a printed outline of the human form, with both front and rear views. Patients are asked to shade in the areas on the figures where they have pain, numbness, or other strange sensations. The Pain Description Scale (see Figure 1.2 on page 17) is simply a horizontal line, with one end marked "1—Least Pos-

Pain Diagram

Please mark the diagram according to the symptoms you are currently experiencing. Indicate the location of your symptoms and the nature of your symptoms by using the markers shown here.

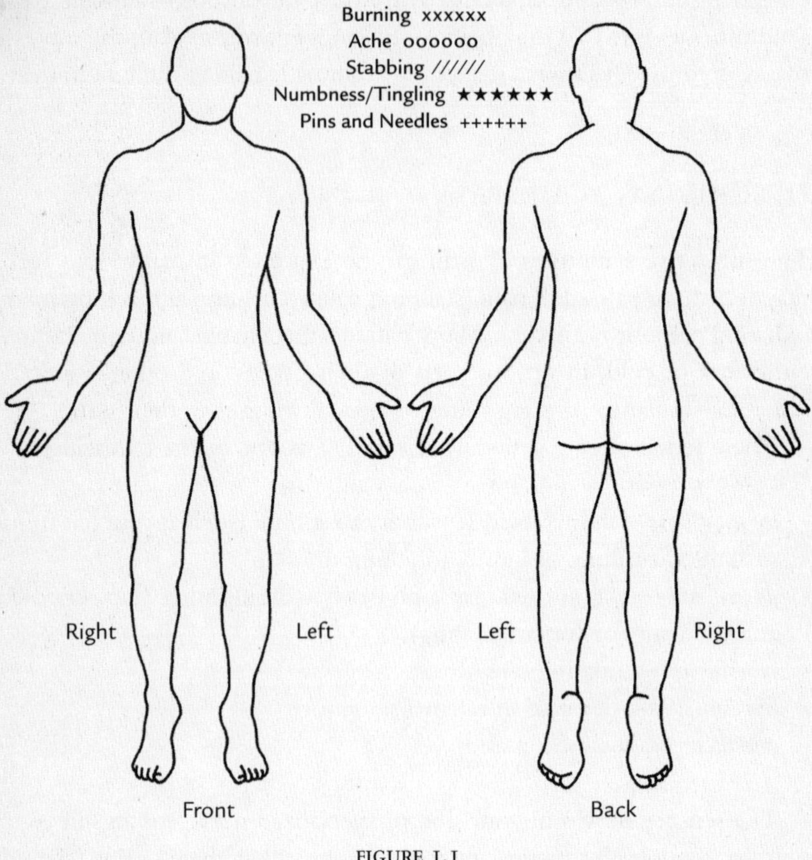

FIGURE I.I

sible Pain," and the other end marked "10—Worst Possible Pain." Patients are asked to place a mark on this scale from one to ten that best describes their overall pain condition.

As you can see, these test figures are just written substitutes for a description of pain. They can give a medical provider a visual picture of the symptoms you are describing. The figures or scales can't diagnose

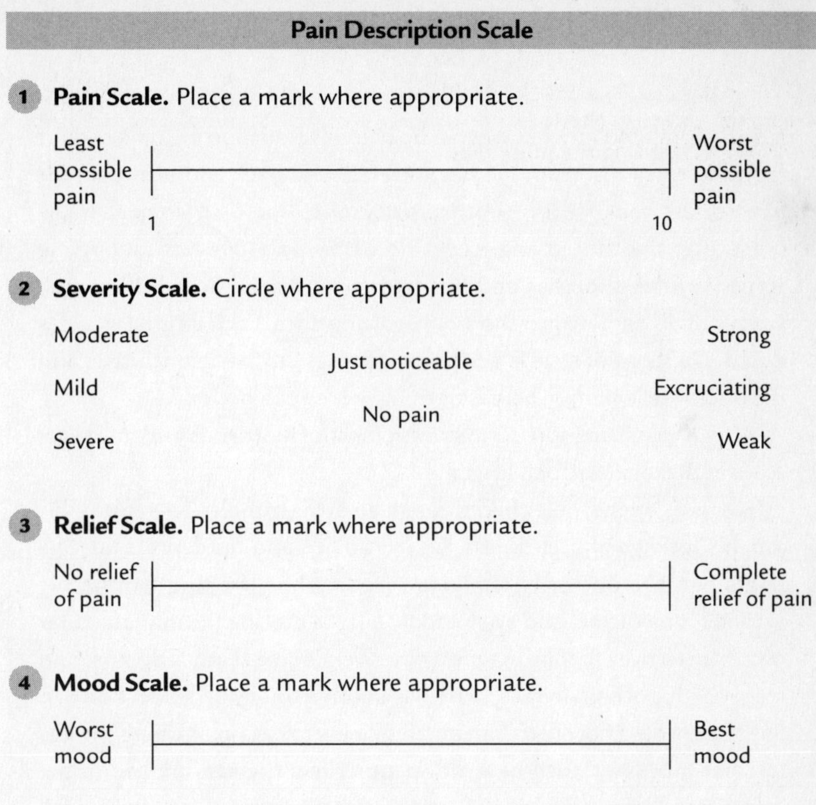

FIGURE 1.2

your condition; they are just another step in a process to determine why you still hurt.

Other tests can be given to determine how you feel about your painful condition. These are longer written tests, usually multiple choice, the answers to which are "graded" by a professionally established scoring procedure, often done by computer.

Standardized written tests such as the Minnesota Multiphasic Personality Inventory (M.M.P.I.) and the Beck Depression Inventory can give your medical provider a greater sense of your emotional status. Unfortunately, you usually do not get to see the results of these tests. The answers are used by those medical providers who are most concerned with your emotional well-being, such as psychologists, psychiatrists, and pain specialists.

A LOSS OF HOPE

Larry was injured at work when a box he was transporting on a forklift fell and struck his head. He has suffered with neck and arm pain for more than a year. He has gone from doctor to doctor, trying one treatment after another, trying to get rid of his pain. He has undergone surgery on his shoulder and has had more than a dozen diagnostic studies of his neck, which show only bulging discs. Each time he changes doctors, a series of tests is performed, the results are inconclusive, and the doctor tells him, "There is nothing more I can do for you."

After a year, Larry lost contact with most of his friends and no longer plays in the local softball league.

His wife, Arlene, helps him through all of his troubles—the loss of his job, his feelings of uselessness, his irritability, and his depression. She treats him like one of her children, feeding him, helping him bathe, getting his medicine, and even finding a lawyer to sue the manufacturer of the "defective" forklift. Arlene aggressively lobbies Larry's doctors and lawyer on his behalf. In fact, Larry has become totally dependent on her. She has devoted her life to him and his illness to the point where she has lost her job. Now they have no income, few friends, and no hope. Arlene cries every night after Larry's numerous pain pills help him fall asleep.

Larry feels out of shape, useless, and depressed. He needs help—but the help must come from within himself. Do you recognize yourself in this story?

BREAKING THE CYCLE OF PAIN

If you suffer from post-traumatic pain syndrome, it can affect your family, your friends, and your coworkers. In fact, the way you cope with your persistent pain affects your entire life. Your marriage may suffer. Children whose mothers or fathers are distracted by pain may develop abnormal behavior. Many coworkers soon tire of filling in for a disabled worker. Bosses may not understand a worker's persistent complaints, limitations, and personality changes, and may fire an injured worker whom they view as being uncooperative. Friends may lose interest in sufferers who complain of persistent pain and may begin to shun them, leaving them even more alone and depressed.

This downward spiral of pain, irritability, depression, physical deconditioning, and isolation can be reversed only when the sufferer throws off the burden of feeling hopeless and dependent. Anyone who suffers from persistent pain must begin to have hope and must gain the motivation to begin to recondition both body and mind. This may require setting new, more realistic goals, while accepting some permanent physical limitations. But this reversal can and must be accomplished.

SUGGESTED READINGS

Galer, B.S. *A Clinical Guide to Neuropathic Pain*. Minneapolis: McGraw-Hill, 2000.

Hooshman, H. *Chronic Pain*. Boca Raton, FL: CRC Press, 1993.

Parsons, D. "Recovery," in *Quantifying Trauma,* vol. 10, no. 1, page 8, Spring 1999.

HELPFUL WEB SITES

American Pain Society
http://www.ampainsoc.org

Centerwatch
http://www.centerwatch.com

Health on the Net Foundation
http://www.hon.ch

2

Hidden-Disc and Referred-Pain Syndromes

WILLIAM H. SIMON, M.D.

Two unusual—but not infrequent—results of trauma can cause chronic pain. These two clinical consequences of trauma are called hidden-disc syndrome (HDS) and referred-pain syndrome (RPS). They may explain your persistent pain.

HIDDEN-DISC SYNDROME

Months ago, you had an accident. You still have pain. You have tried rest, therapy, bracing, and medicine—all kinds of medicine! You may have seen six different doctors—a generalist, a neurologist, a neurosurgeon, an orthopedic surgeon, a doctor of physical medicine, and a psychologist. You may have had X-rays, CAT scans, MRI scans, myelograms, and bone scans, but not one of these fancy, expensive, and sometimes painful tests has been able to determine why you hurt.

You may have been told so many times that there is nothing wrong with you and that the pain is "all in your head" that you are starting to believe it, and that's really frustrating. Has that drunken driver who hit your car made you crazy? Don't lose hope! Many cases of unexplained pain have a reasonable explanation, and it's called hidden-disc syndrome.

You may wonder, "If hidden-disc syndrome is causing my pain, why doesn't my doctor know this?" Doctors are trained to make a diagnosis: to find the cause before they treat a problem. In order to make a diagnosis, your doctor must find something wrong with you that could explain your symptoms—for example, an abnormal X-ray or blood count. If tests show nothing abnormal, your doctor cannot make a diagnosis and therefore can't start treatment. So you may be labeled a chronic complainer, and off you go to another doctor.

Diagnosing hidden-disc syndrome takes time. Multiple examinations are necessary; your doctor has to listen carefully to what you say; and what you say must be relevant, convincing, and consistent. In addition, your doctor must be well grounded in anatomy, physiology (how the body works), and neurology. Most important, your doctor must have empathy: He or she has to be on your wavelength when it comes to your physical complaints. How often does that combination of circumstances take place in today's world of managed care? Unfortunately, not very often.

Even more disturbing than the fact that doctors don't have enough time to diagnose hidden-disc syndrome is the fact that there really are those who have nothing physically wrong with them, despite their complaints. And it is a lot simpler for a doctor to place you in this "nothing wrong" category than it is to make a diagnosis of hidden-disc syndrome—which, incidentally, is not accepted as a diagnosis by all physicians.

Discs are the shock absorbers located between the bones of your spine, your neck (cervical spine), your mid back (thoracic spine), and your low back (lumbar spine). These discs are 80-percent water, and each one has a jellylike center called a nucleus that is surrounded by laminated layers of fibrous tissue. (See Figure 2.1 on page 22.)

These discs have no nerves, but there are plenty of nerve endings around the outside of each disc, and these nerve endings all lead elsewhere. They form nerve roots that exit the spine, neck, chest, and back. These nerve roots come together to form the nerves that carry sensation from all over the body—the head, neck, back, chest, abdomen, arms, and legs. They also supply motor power to all the muscles.

Sometimes a disc is injured in an accident such as a motor-vehicle ac-

Vertebral Disc

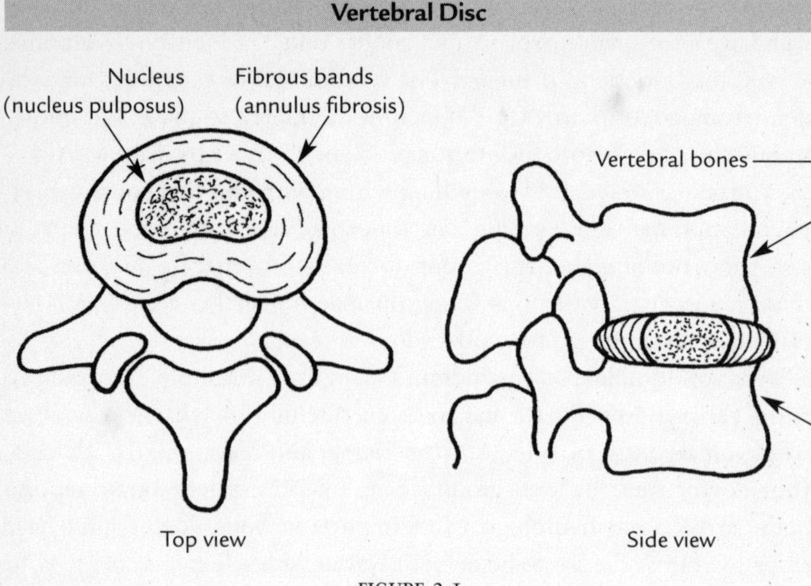

FIGURE 2.1

cident, a work-related injury, or a bad fall. When the force placed on a disc at the time of an injury is more than it can absorb, the disc cracks or tears. If it is a bad tear, the nucleus ruptures out of its central position and enters the spinal canal. This is called a ruptured, or herniated, disc. A herniated disc can cause pain in the neck, arms, back, or legs. A CAT scan, MRI scan, or myelogram can discover a herniated disc, and your doctor can make the diagnosis and begin to treat you. However, if a disc tears but doesn't rupture, your doctor won't find it on any of those tests. Then it becomes the hidden-disc syndrome. The injury is there, and it can cause the same symptoms as a herniated disc, but it is hidden from all the usual diagnostic tests.

Unfortunately, the situation can be even more complicated. Many of us have certain conditions of the spine, which are described below, particularly as we age. These conditions are easily diagnosed and usually don't cause pain. However, they may make you more vulnerable to developing hidden-disc syndrome. These conditions include degenerative joint disease of the spine (spondylitis), degenerative disc disease, spondylolysis, spondylolisthesis, spinal stenosis, and sacralized lumbar vertebra. Each of these conditions has an important relationship to hidden-disc syndrome.

Degenerative Disease of Joints and Discs

As we age, our bodies begin to wear out, and the joints that allow our spine to move in all directions gradually lose their slippery surfaces. Our bodies try to repair this damage but succeed only in producing bone spurs that take up space in the nerve canals of the spine and tend to pinch the nerve roots that exit the spine, neck, mid back, and lower back. A pinched nerve or nerve root can cause pain, weakness, numbness, or an odd sensation that feels like running water, depending upon whether the nerve fibers that are pinched are motor (controlling muscle action) or sensory (controlling sensation). Since the disease process just creeps along, getting progressively worse over the years, a person with this condition may not notice or may dismiss gradual changes in muscle strength or changes in sensation in his or her arms, legs, or trunk. Many people consider these gradual changes to be the natural results of aging when they discover that they can't run as fast or lift as much as they could ten or twenty years earlier.

Moreover, some of us age faster or slower than others. This rate of change mainly depends on how we were genetically put together the

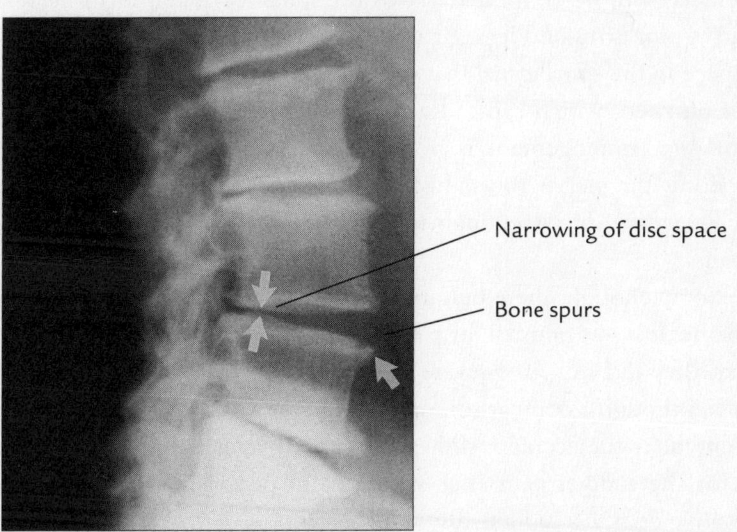

FIGURE 2.2
X-ray showing hallmarks of degenerative disease

moment Dad's sperm met Mom's egg. Some of us inherit strong joints that don't wear out until we are in our sixties or seventies; others of us are genetically programmed to develop wear-and-tear changes, with the development of bone spurs, in our thirties or forties. Most of us over the age of fifty-five have some degenerative joint disease (DJD) of the spine that can be seen easily on X-rays.

Similarly, another condition called degenerative disc disease (DDD) is also strongly influenced by genetic factors. When our intervertebral discs (the shock absorbers between the bones of our spine) wear out, several things happen. First, the shock absorber collapses, and the space between the spinal bones decreases. Next, the disc material bulges around the edges. Think of a tire's partially deflated inner tube; if you were to put pressure on it by jumping on it, it would bulge. Something similar happens to a degenerative disc that is stressed by muscle force or body weight. Again, this wearing-out process occurs slowly, over many years. And, as in the case of arthritis of the spinal joints, some of us develop bulging discs early in life, and some later. By age fifty-five, most of us have bulging discs that can be identified by a CAT scan or an MRI scan.

Any abnormal function of an intervertebral disc can stimulate the many small nerve endings around the outside of a disc. These nerve endings connect with nerve roots that exit the spinal cord and form nerves that lead to our arms and legs. At times, the bulge of a disc takes up so much space in the spinal canal that the nerve roots are actually impinged upon or pinched, which can cause pain or weakness in the back, neck, arms, or legs. Impingement is not even necessary to send abnormal signals along the nerve roots; just an abnormal mechanical function of a degenerative disc is enough to stimulate these nerve endings and cause pain.

Amazingly enough, these bulging degenerative discs don't cause pain in everyone. It is not unusual for patients with this condition to honestly state that they did not have severe spinal pain until after they were injured, even though a comparison of X-rays and other studies made both before and after the accident shows the same images. Often, the explanation for the sudden pain after an injury in people who suffer from degenerative discs is a hidden-disc injury.

Spondylolysis

Spondylolysis refers to a common weakness in a part of the low back (see Figure 2.3 below) that occurs soon after birth. Five percent of us have this defect on one side of the back and never know it—until an X-ray is taken. This defect itself does not cause pain, but it represents a weakness in the low back that can be aggravated by an injury. In other words, if you have a spondylolysis, you are more likely to have hidden-disc syndrome after an injury than someone who has a stronger back.

Spondylolisthesis

Anyone who has two spondylolytic bony defects, one on each side, may develop a condition called spondylolisthesis. In this condition, one bone in the low back (usually the fifth lumbar vertebra) slips forward. The slip may be minor (first-degree), or, in rare cases, the top bone may fall in front of the bottom bone (fifth-degree). In all of these cases, the patient is said to have an unstable low-back condition. (See Figure 2.4 on page 26.)

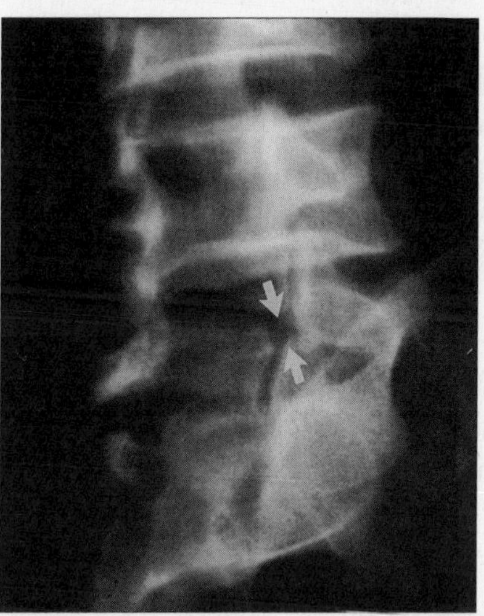

FIGURE 2.3
X-ray showing spondylolysis. Arrows indicate the weak portions of the bone.

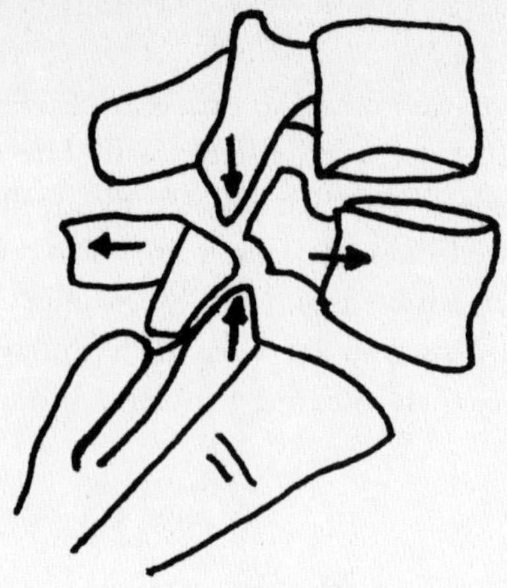

FIGURE 2.4
Spondylolisthesis. Arrows indicate the directions that vertebral bones may slip.

Amazingly enough, most people who have first- or second-degree slips don't know they have the condition. They have backaches like the rest of us. Then, after a fall or an accident, an X-ray is taken, and there it is! Often this condition, which probably has been present since adolescence, is blamed as the cause of all the patient's persistent post-traumatic pain. In many instances, this is simply not true. The spondylolisthesis acts just like the spondylolysis—as a place of least resistance, or a weakness in the low back, which allows a hidden-disc injury to occur at the level above.

Spinal Stenosis

A narrowing of the spinal canal is called spinal stenosis. This narrowing pinches or impinges on those nerve roots that control motion and feeling in our arms and legs. The spinal canal has bony walls that contain those joints that develop degenerative disease with bone spurs. The floor of the canal is the back of the intervertebral disc that bulges in most of us who are more than fifty-five years of age. The combination of the thickening that gradually occurs in the spinal ligaments with age, bony spurs in the joints, and a bulging disc can narrow the spinal canal to the "pinching" point.

Those who are born with smaller spinal canals than others live with so-called congenital (from birth) spinal stenosis all their lives. Many of those who have this condition aren't aware of it until after an accident; until then, they consider the weakness, numbness, or odd sensations that gradually affect their legs to be part of the natural process of growing older.

An X-ray, a CAT scan, or an MRI scan of someone who has spinal stenosis looks bad: There is literally no room for the nerve roots to exit the spinal cord. In reality, these studies would have looked just as bad before the trauma. But a doctor who examines someone who had no pain before an accident may blame the pain on spinal stenosis, when in fact the cause is a subtle hidden-disc injury—a "straw" that literally breaks the patient's back.

Sacralized Lumbar Vertebra

Another condition that could make you vulnerable to hidden-disc syndrome is called a sacralized fifth lumbar vertebra. People with this condition were born with only four moveable bones in their low back (and four intervertebral discs) instead of five. This congenital condition occurs in about 2 percent of people.

When there are only four instead of five shock absorbers, the fourth, or lowest disc, takes a beating and usually undergoes early degenerative disc disease. Anyone who has this condition and who sustains a spinal injury has a greater chance of suffering a hidden-disc injury than someone who has a normal low back.

ADJUSTING TO HIDDEN-DISC INJURIES

Let us look at three clinical examples of patients who have experienced hidden-disc syndrome and have learned to live with it.

Ann is a thirty-two-year-old attorney. When she stopped her car at a traffic light, another car plowed into the rear of her car. Since then, she has suffered with neck and upper-back pain accompanied by numbness that radiates into both arms. Her neck X-rays showed some mild arthritis. An MRI scan confirmed that she has mild arthritis but no disc herniation. Her physical exam demonstrated only mild pain in the back of her neck. She tried physical therapy, pain medicine, and a cervical collar, but she still could not do her work as an attorney because of the pain. And she really wanted to work; a prestigious law firm had just hired her, and she wanted to keep her position. Ultimately, after several months of treatment, she had to compromise. She reduced her lifting, limited her reading and writing to shorter periods of time, and arranged to work only part time. With these limitations on stressing her injured but hidden cervical disc, she continues to function and do the work she loves.

Michael, a forty-nine-year-old driver of a cement truck, was knocked down by his truck's cement chute while pouring cement. He has suffered with pain in his low back and down his left leg for more than a year. He cannot stand or sit for any length of time without the recurrence of pain. His MRI scan showed that he has severe spinal stenosis, with degenerative joint disease in his low back (despite his relatively young age). Ultimately, a surgeon operated on his spine to give his nerve roots more room. He did get some relief from pain, but physical findings continue to indicate that his lumbar nerve roots were injured. In other words, his spinal stenosis was relieved, but his hidden-disc injury remains. He will not be able to return to his previous occupation, but if he is motivated enough, he will be able to return to work in a more sedentary job.

Helen is a sixty-two-year-old medical secretary who tripped and fell down a flight of stairs. For two years, she suffered recurrent pain in the back of her neck radiating into her right shoulder. X-rays of her neck showed degenerative joint disease and degenerative disc disease at four disc spaces in her neck, although no disc herniation was found on her MRI scan. She admits to having had occasional aches and pains in her neck and right shoulder before the accident, but nothing as severe as the pain she felt after the fall. She is able to work, despite her hidden-disc injury, but has to depend on exercises, a special pillow, and over-the-counter medicine to keep going. But she keeps going!

So what can you do if you have hidden-disc syndrome? Occasionally, surgery is the answer if hidden-disc syndrome is associated with spinal stenosis or spondylolisthesis. More often, you will have to learn to change your lifestyle—and the second part of this book will help you.

In the meantime, at least you will know that there is a real cause of your pain. Read on.

REFERRED-PAIN SYNDROME

Strana citta! the Italians cry—"weird city," or "very strange." That phrase describes referred-pain syndrome (RPS). With this condition, you feel pain in one part of your body, but the cause of the pain is in another part. For example, after an injury, your knee hurts, but you have fractured your hip. Or your shoulder hurts, but you have ruptured a disc in your neck. Or your foot hurts, but you have injured your low back.

Not only is this condition hard for you to accept, but it is also frequently overlooked by very well-meaning physicians. So, too often, treatment to the wrong area continues without relief. Often surgery is tried, to no avail, and the patient continues to be in pain, all because no one realizes that the origin of the pain is elsewhere.

How can our bodies send us such misleading signals? As the brain interprets signals from the central nervous system, it does not always distinguish between signals at the origin of the injury and signals at connecting locations. For example, a distribution of nerve roots coming out of our spinal cord sensitizes certain areas of the skin. (See Figure 2.5 on page 30.) Within this pattern, to take just one example, nerve roots that supply nerves to the skin of the thigh (L5) also supply nerves to skin on the calf and foot. Therefore, an injury to the lower spine may be felt as pain in the hip, knee, or foot.

As Figure 2.5 shows, nerves from the cervical spine serve the head, jaw, shoulders, chest, elbows, wrists, and fingers, so an injury to the cervical spine may cause pain in any of these areas. Nerves from the thoracic spine (mid back) serve the chest and abdomen, and nerves from the lumbar spine (low back) run to the groin, hips, knees, calves, ankles, and toes.

To make diagnosis even more difficult, in many cases there is an actual injury to the site of the referred pain. Imagine a fractured tibia (lower leg) and a lower-spine injury occurring together. The pain of the leg fracture focuses the patient's attention on this injured limb throughout the healing process. Then, even months after the leg has healed, the patient falsely perceives that the pain from the fracture is still present because of referred pain from the injured spine. This patient has post-traumatic pain syndrome caused by referred pain.

Referred pain may affect any part of your body, from head to toe. Headache may be the result of an injury to the upper cervical spine. Persistent pain in the elbow (often called tennis elbow even in patients who

The Spinal Nerves and Where They Go in the Body

C=Cervical, Th=Thoracic, L=Lumbar, S=Sacral

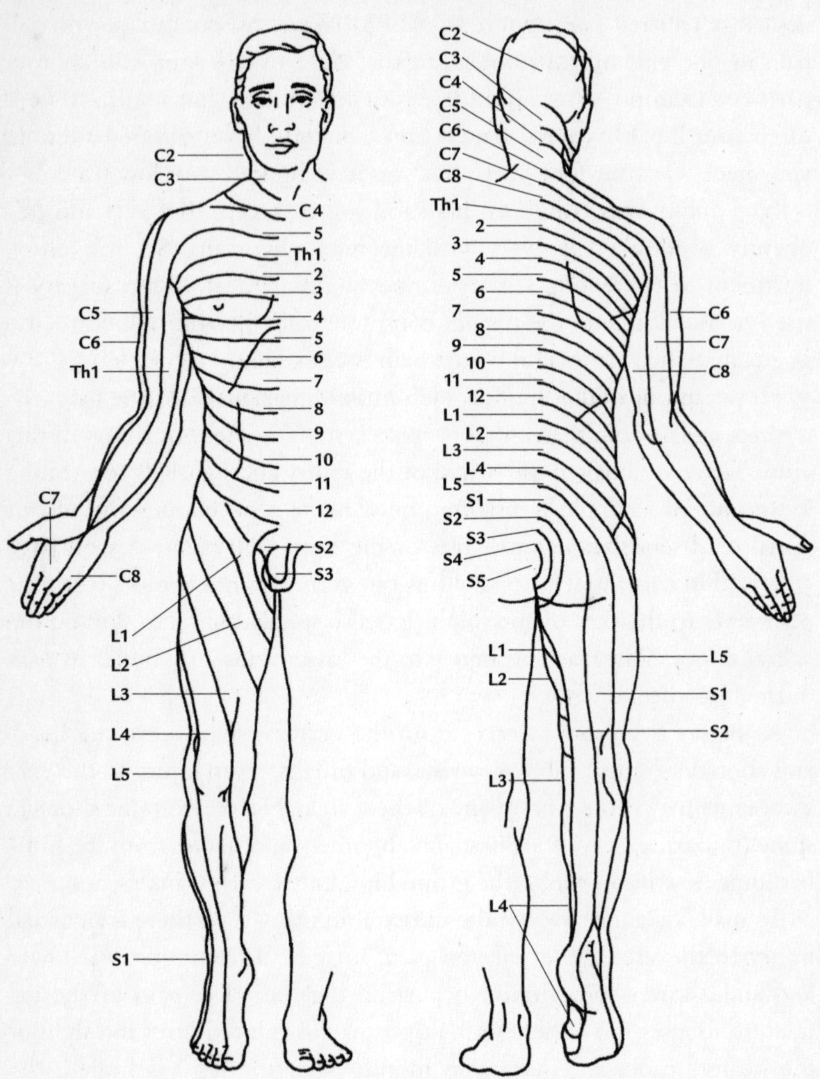

FIGURE 2.5

The spinal nerves and the corresponding areas of the body that they affect.

don't play tennis) also may be the result of an injury to the cervical spine. Jaw problems, particularly with the temporomandibular joint, may occur because of a cervical nerve-root injury. Wrist pain, which often is called post-traumatic carpal-tunnel syndrome, may in fact be due to a cervical-disc injury. Finger pain and numbness, often in the fourth and fifth fingers, which is usually thought to be caused by an ulnar nerve injury at the elbow, may be referred from the neck. Chest pain, often confused with symptoms of a heart attack, and abdominal pain, often confused with a serious abdominal problem, both may be due to an injured cervical or thoracic disc. Groin pain, often mistaken for a hernia, as well as hip pain, often confused with joint arthritis, may be the result of low-back trauma. Calf pain that is actually caused by a lumbar-disc injury often is mistaken for phlebitis. Ankle pain may be due to injuries to nerve roots in the lower back that weaken muscles near the joint and that cause recurrent sprains. Pain in the heel may be attributed to a "heel spur" shown on an X-ray, and surgery may be performed on the foot. In fact, this heel pain may be the result of S1 nerve-root irritation.

Many patients who develop referred-pain syndrome after trauma have preexisting spinal conditions with no prior symptoms. These conditions include degenerative disc disease, degenerative joint disease, spondylolisthesis, and spinal stenosis. All of these conditions predispose a patient to subclinical nerve-root irritation—irritation that is present, even though the patient doesn't notice it. After an injury to the spine, this nerve-root irritation may become noticeable, and its origin may fool you since the pain is referred from the spine to another area of the body, such as the arms or legs.

Diabetes mellitus affects the circulation to nerve roots and peripheral nerves, so it also can make these structures more vulnerable to the effects of even relatively minor trauma—and, of course, to the onset of referred pain.

Be Alert to Your Symptoms

It is important that you understand the concept of referred pain. If, for example, you focus on your shoulder discomfort instead of a lesser dysfunction in your neck, you may actually prevent your doctor from treating the proper injured area. Your doctor should be aware of referred-pain syndrome, but if you keep saying, "It's my shoulder! It's my shoulder!"

you may get attention paid to your shoulder and even undergo surgery, when in fact you need attention paid to your injured neck.

Often, once a patient understands the concept of RPS, that person can refocus on the actual area of injury. Then the patient declares, "Oh yes, doctor, my neck does hurt." Surprisingly, once that recognition occurs, the pain in the referred site—shoulder, hand, hip, or knee—becomes less noticeable. That's just how the brain works.

The following are three clinical examples of referred-pain syndrome:

Dolores was thirty-seven years old when she was injured in an automobile accident. She suffered two fractured bones in her right foot. When her cast was removed, her pain persisted. On the theory that the bones had not completely healed, her foot was operated on, but the surgery did not relieve her pain. A year later, upon examination, her doctor found evidence of lumbar nerve-root irritation. An EMG confirmed nerve-root irritation, and an MRI demonstrated a right-sided disc herniation at L5-S1. An operation on her low back removed the herniated disc, and after a period of healing and rehabilitation, she resumed all of her normal daily activities without any pain.

David, a thirty-seven-year-old steelworker, developed severe pain in his hand after striking a piece of steel with a heavy hammer. He underwent two operations on his wrist without any relief from his pain, which prevented him from working. Two years later, an X-ray of his neck revealed degenerative disc disease. An EMG showed left-sided cervical nerve-root irritation. After the referred-pain syndrome from his neck to his hand was explained to him and he was given a neck-care program to maintain for life, he found work that was less physically demanding and he needed no further treatment.

Edith, at age fifty-eight, fell and dislocated her right elbow. The dislocation was reduced, but she continued to complain of such severe pain in her right wrist and thumb that she could not pick up any object with her right hand. X-rays of her hand and wrist were normal, but a X-ray of her neck revealed degenerative disc disease at C5-C6. An MRI scan of her neck showed bulging discs at C3-C4, C4-C5, and C5-C6. When she was treated conservatively with traction and exercises for her bulging cervical discs, she obtained considerable relief from the pain in her wrist and thumb.

Be alert to each of your own symptoms. If you think that your pain might be caused by hidden-disc syndrome or referred-pain syndrome, bring this up with your doctor—and get on the right track to the station known as "relief."

SUGGESTED READINGS

Crock, H.V. "Internal Disc Disruption," in *Practice of Spinal Surgery,* pp. 35–55. Wien, NY: Springer-Verlag, 1983.

Flatman, J.G. "Hip Disease with Referred Pain to the Knee," *Journal of the American Medical Association* 1975 Dec 1; 234(9):967–8.

Hockaday, J.M., et al. "Patterns of Referred Pain in the Normal Subject," *Brain* 1967 Sep; 90(3):481–96.

Hooshmand, H. "Referred Pain and Trigger Point" in *Chronic Pain,* pp. 83–90, CRC Press, Boca Raton, 1993.

Simon, W.H., Ehrlich, G.E. "Spinal Root Pain Referred to Peripheral Areas of Skeletal Injury" in *Medicolegal Consequences of Trauma,* pp. 61–129. New York: Marcel Dekker, 1993.

Vecchiet, L., et al. "Referred Muscle Pain," *Current Review of Pain* 1999; 3(6):489–98.

HELPFUL WEB SITES

Mayo Clinic
http://www.mayohealth.org

National Institutes of Health
http://www.nih.gov/health

National Library of Medicine
http://www.nlm.nih.gov

3

Fibromyalgia, Chronic Pain, and Fatigue

GEORGE E. EHRLICH, M.D.

Just about everyone experiences pain frequently, perhaps even daily. Some pain, such as a deep cut or a severe burn, is acute, or intense, but the pain ultimately abates. Often, pain is transient, or passes quickly, and is not very threatening—a stitch in the side, a stubbed toe, a crick in the neck after a nap, or a twinge in the back after unusual exertion. Pain is, after all, nature's way of calling our attention to something we should not be doing. It's a valuable defense mechanism that keeps us from enacting worse sequels to these activities. These pains don't threaten us; we know what seems to cause or initiate them.

Other pains warn that you've been overdoing some activity, perhaps by doing it too long (such as an athletic event you were reluctant to quit), or by overestimating its difficulty (trying to lift something too heavy), or by repeating the same movement too many times (during prolonged computer keyboarding or knitting). These also result in pain, and this pain doesn't go away so easily, although it, too, will subside if you're patient. We call the events that provoke these pains by a number of names—strains, sprains, charley horses, and so on—and we expect that we'll get over them. Doctors call such pains "subacute": That is, they aren't transient, but they will go away in a reasonable time. Whe matter of hours or days (or, in the case of back pain, even good news is that these pains are not here to stay. Also, the not very severe. But when pains linger, and their discomfort prevents you from sleeping soundly, and you wake up every day realizing that they're still there, they become harder to bear. When these pains become prolonged for three months or more, they are called "chronic pain." Pain is tiring, and when it persists, it leads to fatigue.

We define pain by its severity, its duration, its location, and its repetition. An ache at a joint might suggest arthritis (*arthr-* refers to the joint, and *-itis* means "inflammation"). Even a slight pain in the chest or left shoulder, radiating into the arm and occurring without known provocation, might be cause for worry, as it may signal a heart attack. We sometimes ask for a doctor's advice because such pains are perceived as threatening: "Arthritis? A heart attack? What is it, and what will become of me?" Yet some severe pains, such as toothaches, are often ignored for a while because we think they can't lead to anything worse and that maybe the pain relievers we buy at the supermarket will suffice and spare us a trip to the dentist. So our perception of pain, our interpretation of it, and its timing help determine how we react to it.

The ready availability of pain-relieving medicines and ointments on the shelves of neighborhood stores and the abundance of herbal and other alternative treatments offered by health-food stores and nonmedical practitioners confirm that pain is common. This also reassures us that most other people share our problems with pain. However, this wasn't always the case.

A HISTORY OF PAIN

In the remote past, pain was accepted as part of the human condition. Religious people in many cultures assumed that God had placed humans on earth to suffer and would provide rewards in the afterlife. The ancients often depicted pain: It is described in the Bible, and it is an essential element of *The Iliad* and *The Odyssey;* it can be found in the plays of Sophocles and Euripides and in sculptures such as the ancient Greek sculpture of Laocoön, whose contorted face and body express his suffering. But often such pain was thought to be a result of God's will, intended as punishment for transgressions or for displeasing the one God of the Bible or the pantheon of the Greeks. Pain depicted in these theatrical settings tended to be heroic and acute, and the cause was apparent. For example, the sea serpents tightly coiled around the body of Laocoön clearly cause his pain. In these dramatizations, pain afflicts the noble or ennobles them; chronic pain was generally ignored by ancient sculptors and scribes. In medieval Europe, the bearing of pain by ordinary folk was a religious concept, and even crucifixion paintings portrayed passive acceptance of pain.

At the beginning of the sixteenth century, Hieronymous Bosch painted graphic scenes of tortured souls in hell, but it took Renaissance artists to depict the pain of the gruesome punishment of crucifixion. Not until 1893 did Edvard Munch create what is perhaps the best depiction of a reaction to chronic pain in his famous painting of a face distorted in a scream. So your pain, whether acute or subacute, has historical precedent.

Until recently, the legacy of the past continued to consign the condition of chronic pain to religion. One reason may well have been that no effective means of controlling pain were available, and the intensity of chronic pain was generally less than acute. Cause and effect, too, were only dimly understood; when something preceded the pain, it was assumed to be the cause. The realization that pain is experienced by the mind if inflicted on the body was slow to gain acceptance.

NAMING YOUR PAIN

Chronic pain differs from acute and subacute pain in more than duration; it also differs in its intensity and in what it means to you.

If you have chronic pain, your pain has settled in. Your whole body may hurt, you wake up feeling tired, and fatigue plagues your days. Nothing seems to help; even the distractions of a TV comedy or time off from work afford only temporary relief at best. You probably remember a trauma—that is, an injury—in your recent past. Perhaps your car was rear-ended, and although you felt fine at the time (other than being angry about the damage), you woke up the next morning with a stiff neck and other pains. And they're still there! Or you may have stumbled over a crack in the sidewalk or slipped on the freshly mopped floor of the market, causing you to fall or clumsily cling to a nearby prominence, temporarily skewing your posture.

It may be that whatever injury you sustained has long ago ceased to trouble you, but now generalized pain and fatigue are with you constantly. You consult a physician, who gives your symptoms a name: "fibromyalgia," or perhaps "chronic fatigue syndrome." Before, you had pain; now you have a name for it. Today you can find activist groups, also known as support groups, for people with these diagnoses, and even lawyers who will offer to help you obtain compensation for your suffering.

Does it help to give your pain and fatigue a name? A poem by Anthony Trollope advises:

Nor bring . . .
Some doctor, full of phrase and fame,
To shake his sapient head and give
The ill he cannot cure a name.

Fibromyalgia is a fairly recent name given to generalized chronic pain that is often accompanied by weakness, fatigue, self-perceived memory loss, and constipation or "irritable bowel." None of these symptoms can be verified by a doctor: When you report that they occur, your doctor may choose whether to believe you. But there are no tests to confirm your symptoms, other than to test for excessive tenderness at eighteen points on the body that have been identified as being inordinately tender in cases of fibromyalgia. As it happens, these eighteen spots are tender in everyone, whether or not they are in pain, but when they are touched by an examiner who is looking for fibromyalgia, and when they are registered as being tender, they are said to confirm the diagnosis. This is an example of circular reasoning.

Now you must understand this about medical terms: They are a form of shorthand that permits doctors to talk with one another without having to detail all the symptoms (what you report) and signs (what the examination discloses) each time. Fibromyalgia—which literally means "pain of the fibrous tissues that bind the body together"—is just one of those terms. It describes your symptoms, but not their cause. This concept is often misunderstood, even by doctors, and quite often by support groups.

CHRONIC PAIN BY OTHER NAMES

Over time, chronic pain and fatigue have been known by many names. These include fibrositis, which means "inflammation of the fibrous tissues" (there is no such condition); neurasthenia, which means "nervous weakness"; or one of a host of other descriptive but essentially meaningless terms. Other such names for chronic pain over time include the following:

- chronic appendicitis (which doesn't exist but was, nevertheless, once commonly diagnosed, leading to unjustified appendectomies in which no abnormalities of the appendix could be demonstrated).
- spinal abnormalities, a diagnosis common at the turn of the nineteenth century, which prompted manipulation treatments by chiropractors and even osteopaths.
- peculiar neuralgic affection of females, a diagnosis popular early in the twentieth century.
- insanity, thought to be a result of uterine disease (the word "hysteria" is based on the Greek syllable for uterus, *hyster*), a diagnosis that resulted in many unnecessary hysterectomies.
- reflex abnormalities, nervous exhaustion, and other terms, for which referrals to neurologists and psychiatrists became customary.

All these erroneous concepts were discredited long ago, each one a successor to the theories of demonic possession and witchcraft that prevailed several hundred years earlier.

That the mind interprets pain and participates in its perception should be a truism, but the concept of a connection between body and mind has been resisted again and again.

The concept of psychological participation in pain is considered unacceptable by many people. For this reason, psychological symptoms observed in soldiers during World War I were labeled "shell shock," and because that term implies an organic disorder—a physical impact upon the brain—it became acceptable. In World War II, the term "war neuroses" was sometimes substituted, and although that term more closely defines the symptoms and their causes, it also became unacceptable to many, again because it seemed to suggest a cause that was not strictly physical (although it's hard to understand why someone confronted with the possibility of being maimed or killed should react only physically). This refusal to acknowledge psychologically induced pain is the mindset that led General George Patton to confront a traumatized soldier who had been evacuated from the front to a military hospital and slap him as a weakling worthy of disgust. But pain that results from a psychiatric disorder is not invalid: It is real pain, and it causes real suffering.

SEARCHING FOR A CAUSE

During the twentieth century, the search for infectious causes of chronic pain and fatigue became popular in medical circles in hopes that research might reveal a treatable disease. One such candidate was brucellosis, a disease caused by microbes that reside in sheep and can be transmitted to shepherds. Brucellosis is relatively uncommon in humans, and occurs predominantly in Iceland and other areas of northern Europe; it has never been epidemic. Because fibromyalgia is diagnosed far more often in whites than in any other race, the correlation of patients who had chronic pain with patients of northern European heritage seemed to make some sense, and as a result, brucellosis was popularly, and incorrectly, overdiagnosed some fifty or sixty years ago.

When brucellosis was disproved as a cause of fibromyalgia, lupus erythematosus took its place for a time as a potential cause for the same set of symptoms. This disease does exist and can be legitimately diagnosed and confirmed by laboratory data. It is often accompanied by chronic pain, and in the 1960s and 1970s it became a vogue diagnosis, like all those listed above, for many people who clearly did not manifest the disease of lupus. More recently, Lyme disease, another infectious disease, has been vastly overdiagnosed and overtreated.

In each case, even an incorrect diagnosis and overtreatment were acceptable to those who preferred to find some external cause for their maladies. Our lives follow a sequence, the present following the past, the future before us. This means that many events succeed each other in time. Often, we think that because one event came first and another later, they must somehow be related, one causing the other. This concept is embodied in the Latin saying, *post hoc, ergo propter hoc:* "After this, therefore because of this." But the only relationship between two events may be their position in the sequence, one preceding and the other following. It may seem logical to conclude that the first event caused the second, but analysis may show no connection other than position in time.

Many misconceptions can arise when an individual becomes convinced that one event causes a later event. Silicone breast implants are one such example: When millions of women chose to have this procedure, you would expect that they would experience the normal range of events that would occur in any such large group—that some would develop generalized pains, some would develop arthritis, and some would experience other disorders. If these women had not shared a common event, such as the implant, the occurrence of the disorders that followed would not provoke comment, as it followed the pattern that occurs in any population of this size. But because these women shared the common experience of a breast implant, many of them became convinced that their implants caused their later disorders. They could not be dissuaded of this relationship, and many appeared on talk shows or were quoted in the media as saying, "I am the evidence." Carefully conducted studies overwhelmingly disprove this causal relationship, but these studies fail to persuade many women who still believe that what came first must be responsible for what followed.

Similarly, even today, the popular media have convinced many that the Epstein-Barr virus causes fibromyalgia, even though this virus is ubiquitous, or widespread, and most people will show exposure to it if given a blood test. But this virus is not the agent that causes the pains.

Chronic pains that have no apparent cause need names, and these names have been given, in a progression from an apparent understanding of cause to today's acknowledgment of uncertain cause. Contemporary labels for chronic pain and fatigue derive from these conflicting and conflicted views. When pain predominates, we call it fibromyalgia; when fatigue or weakness is the primary symptom, we call it chronic fatigue syndrome, using the word "syndrome" to describe the sum total of similar symptoms reported by patients.

These terms sound ominous, and they encompass symptoms that reduce the quality of life: Work and play are difficult, and sometimes they are insurmountable obstacles. Concentrating on these symptoms interferes with most pleasures, even sex. When a thorough medical examination and lots of expensive and often unpleasant tests fail to reveal a cause, it's frustrating. When the doctor can't find anything, you may seek out another doctor and go through all this again, or you may find a support group that brings you together with others who are similarly frustrated.

People who have such symptoms as chronic fatigue and pain often become hostile toward their doctors out of frustration; this only makes doctors respond in kind, which doesn't help. The doctors also may be frustrated; they accept that you have pain, but they don't know how to help you. They don't want to suggest that it's all in your mind—and it isn't—or that some environmental, social, or psychological factors may play a part in it. For many patients, a psychological explanation, even if it's only a part of the cause, is perceived as criticism; it's as if the medical establishment doesn't believe that you're suffering.

SEARCHING FOR A CURE

You may have found that the medication prescribed for you hasn't helped, nor have the remedies suggested by your neighbor. You may still sleep poorly and wake up tired and listless. It may seem that your world has no color. And then you come across an article in a newspaper or magazine, or someone directs you to a book that features the name the doctor gave your pains and fatigue: fibromyalgia and chronic fatigue syndrome. These articles usually are addressed to women, and in fact most people who complain of these symptoms are women. National organizations such as the Arthritis Foundation publish pamphlets on the subject of fibromyalgia and chronic fatigue syndrome, and daytime talk shows feature guests who tell the same story. So doesn't that disprove any suggestion that these symptoms have some psychological basis? No.

Your pain is real enough, and so is your fatigue. No one can deny your suffering, and no one else can feel your pain, except symbolically. As has already been pointed out, specialized parts of your body produce the pain, but your mind recognizes it, interprets it, and sometimes even causes it.

While most pains end of their own accord, chronic pain develops when substances that the body releases at the site of the original acute pain alter receptors in the spinal cord and the brain so that they become more sensitive to pain. Among these substances are prostaglandins, the same molecules that anti-inflammatory drugs are meant to suppress. Prostaglandins cause the initial swelling of damaged tissues and sensitize the nerve endings. Normally, they become inactive when their job is done, but sometimes the changes they have wrought persist. It is these persistent symptoms that we call chronic pain, and, unfortunately, unjustifiable names have been attached to them.

To reject the term "fibromyalgia" is not to minimize your pain or to suggest you are malingering or making it all up. But the term should be rejected, because it leads nowhere and won't help you find a solution. Yes, your accident or other trauma may have initiated the problem, but dwelling on your anger and your pain aggravates it, and the seeming indifference of others (perhaps someone near to you, or perhaps your doctor) increases not only your frustration but also the severity of your symptoms.

Letting pain govern your life—focusing on it and letting it take over, to exclude your loved ones, your coworkers, and your neighbors, or allowing it to become so central that you can think and talk of nothing else—only makes matters worse. Studies have confirmed that such behavior ultimately leads to social isolation and exclusion, producing all the consequences we hope to avoid. Others' sympathy may turn to avoidance, and pain can become a self-fulfilling prophecy: "Why am I alone? Why can't someone help?"

Litigation prolongs the discomfort by forcing you to prove that you hurt, prove that you can't function normally. You will be sent to doctors who will label you as a fraud or a financial opportunist. A series of examinations and hearings may gain you Social Security disability compensation, but it may come at the cost of your self-respect. And that hoped-for financial reward may not help you get well if you should become caught up in what the wise rheumatologist Nortin Hadler has called the "disability vortex."

So is it hopeless? By no means.

HOPE

Long ago, it was said that it's not enough to add years to life without adding life to years. Chapter 8 will describe what works and what doesn't to help you improve. In the meantime, it's important not to get hung up on the diagnosis. Certainly, when an infection causes pneumonia, we can identify the cause; when a blood clot or narrowing in an artery results in a heart attack, we understand the process. But when it comes to pains that have no apparent cause, we share with others the bafflement that the pain produces.

Earlier, we observed that everyone has some pain some of the time. In a lifetime, everyone probably experiences some chronic pain, too. What we do with this pain, how we deal with it, and what it means to us become important in understanding and treating it.

Perception of pain and response to it varies from individual to individual and from culture to culture. In many rural communities, and in many cultures, complaining of pain is unacceptable. Those who have it get on with their lives, as complaining would do no good. In urbanized societies, especially in North America and Europe, advanced medical-care systems recognize and attempt to treat pain, and insurances policies and governments even offer compensation to the sufferers. The anonymity of big cities, the relative difficulty of defining one's place in these societies, and the displacement of basic values all collaborate to turn small pains into big pains. You've seen the commercials or read the labels: "For minor pains [of arthritis or whatever], take . . ." To the sufferer, there are no minor pains. If you perceive enough pain to want to do something about it, it's not minor to you.

Please recognize that you share your pain with all of humanity, and the event that may seem to have caused it (or which others claim caused it) might only have brought it to your attention. Forget the names fibromyalgia and chronic fatigue syndrome. They are meaningless, even if your symptoms aren't.

Your symptoms are treatable. Life can again become enjoyable, and the gloom and doom can be made to dissipate. You are not condemned to an earthbound purgatory, and you are not different from your neighbors. Your symptoms may be more severe on the scale that encompasses all of us, but you can overcome them.

The presumption on the part of patients and their physicians that an organic trauma or disease is the only legitimate cause of symptoms has led to a current overinvestigation of the symptoms. It also has led patients to assume a "sick role" that has been thrust on them, as the Canadian rheumatologist Anthony Russell avers, by sympathetic physicians.

This concept also has fostered a veritable hotbed of research seeking organic factors, both internal and external, that precipitate the symptoms and implicate trauma as a cause.

Almost every "finding" trumpeted by the media to explain the manifestations of chronic pain and fatigue has been either disproven or shown to be so common as to be shared by the majority of the general population. For example, although some have linked sleeping abnormalities and changes in weather to symptoms of fatigue and pain, these experiences are also shared by those who don't have the symptoms, and may turn out to be nonspecific. How is that possible? One explanation is the concept that statisticians call bias, which prejudices the results of studies that include those who complain of disorders and exclude those who don't.

So forget the names for your symptoms, and move on with your life. Remember: The only differences between chronic pain and the terms fibromyalgia and chronic fatigue syndrome are the names we give to our distress, our perception of it, and our reaction to it. Without these terms, without the so-called support systems, and without the medicalization of the pains—that is, agreement by doctors, lawyers, support groups, and some disability compensation systems that the name "fibromyalgia" somehow defines a different entity and that therefore this entity is more harmful—you would gradually feel better and be able to resume normal activities sooner. When you accept these labels, improvement is difficult: Too many vested interests want to keep you disabled and unhappy for their own (sometimes even well-meaning) purposes.

How then do fibromyalgia and chronic fatigue syndrome differ from chronic pain in general? They are named, and their names instill fear, and they spread like infectious diseases, through word of mouth and through professional and popular literature. As these names amplify and publicize the symptoms, they become fixed in "conventional wisdom." The physical symptoms are then augmented by a mental state that helps to stimulate—as a consequence, not as a cause—molecular substances that help prolong the pain.

Fibromyalgia and chronic fatigue syndrome are no different from other chronic pain; they only appear to be different. Once you accept this, you will see that you don't have some chronic, disabling disorder. And when you realize this, you can begin to reclaim your health.

SUGGESTED READINGS

Arthritis Today

A magazine published bimonthly by the Arthritis Foundation, which is also available online at http://www.arthritis.org/resources/. (One caveat: Its articles, written by science writers, tend to support the diagnosis without getting to the fact that these symptoms are shared by those who are afflicted as well as those who are not.)

Showalter, Elaine. *Hystories: Hysterical Epidemics and Modern Media.* New York: Columbia University Press, 1997.

This readable exposition, available in a trade paperback edition, explains how the term "chronic fatigue syndrome" and, by extrapolation, the closely related term "fibromyalgia" gained currency and can mislead.

4

Hidden Concussions

ARNOLD SADWIN, M.D.

Each year, millions of people suffer head injuries that set off a chain reaction of physical and emotional symptoms, including pain, sleep disturbances, fatigue, loss of concentration, and depression. A head injury can cause more than three dozen other symptoms, and physicians usually describe any group of these symptoms as post-concussion syndrome (PCS).

A cerebral concussion takes place when a jolt or a blow forces the gelatinous brain to bump against the hard protective covering of the skull. A sudden, jarring impact can cause a concussion even if you do not hit your head against another object and even if you remain conscious.

A concussion is like a "brain quake," and it usually causes a momentary altered state of awareness, a *dysconscious* episode. This has been described as "having your bell rung" or receiving a "ding," especially in contact sports. Athletes often describe seeing stars or a flash of light at the moment of impact. Some recover quickly, and others experience lingering symptoms.

Most concussions are caused by motor-vehicle accidents, falls, or sports injuries. In recent years, more attention is being paid to students and professional athletes who have been stunned during a game. The examination of injured athletes is becoming more stringent, but in the past, athletes were allowed to go back into the game too soon, making them more susceptible to subsequent head trauma. Eric Lindros, the legendary hockey star, and Troy Aikman, the champion quarterback, have each suffered much-publicized concussions, reminding all of us of the inherent danger in contact sports. In boxing, the goal is to give your opponent a concussion. These repeated head injuries eventually take their toll; Muhammad Ali, who may have had more concussions than any other person, has developed post-traumatic Parkinson's disease.

Although it's easy to recognize the seriousness of severe sports injuries, some concussions are more subtle. Violently shaking an infant or child can cause permanent brain damage, or even death, from a set of injuries known as "shaken baby syndrome." More commonly, a child at play may suffer a slight concussion without realizing it and may develop temporary symptoms. An adult who unknowingly receives a concussion may develop permanent problems. A child's brain is more resilient and therefore may recover more quickly and completely.

ONE CAUSE OF MANY PROBLEMS

This chapter describes hidden concussions, whether undiagnosed or misdiagnosed, and explains why many painful physical and emotional problems occur and persist.

It's possible to have a cerebral concussion without realizing it. How could this happen? Any event that severely shakes your head and jars the soft brain tissue against the bony skull can tear microscopic fibers and significantly injure some of the billions of nerve cells and fibers that you use for mental activity.

For example, what if you were in a motor-vehicle accident and were shaken up but had not hit your head? You might sit motionless, holding the steering wheel, unaware of the passage of time. You could be dazed momentarily or for an extended length of time. Later, you might develop any of forty or more symptoms as a result of your injury, without knowing the cause. You might have persistent pain as well as changes in your personality and thinking ability. You might become so forgetful that you could become concerned that you are developing early Alzheimer's disease.

A CASE IN POINT: ONE MISSTEP

A fifty-year-old woman fractured her ankle when she stepped out of her four-wheel-drive vehicle onto an unstable two-by-four board at a construction site. She was treated for a broken ankle, but she continued to have pain long after the break healed, and became depressed. For years her pain and depression continued, despite treatment. Psychotherapy did not appreciably relieve her emotional problems, and her depression was blamed on the continual pain in her ankle, which caused her to use a cane. She and her orthopedist wondered why she was not improving, and eventually she became so depressed that she made three suicide attempts.

Eleven years after her accident, her psychiatrist referred her to a neuropsychiatrist who specializes in post-concussion syndrome. On taking her initial history, he realized that she had had about a five-second loss of awareness at the time of her injury. She remembered stepping down from her vehicle but had no recollection of falling or twisting her ankle. She next recalled getting up and noticing that her ankle was painful and swollen. Later, she remembered feeling a painful jolt from her ankle to her leg and into her back, and finally into her head.

Her neuropsychiatrist found that she had nearly all of the symptoms of post-concussion syndrome, including hallucinations and seizures. She was given appropriate medications and soon experienced considerable relief from her symptoms. Later, after utilizing faith healing, she no longer needed a cane. This is an unusual example of a missed diagnosis that was eventually suspected by a psychiatrist and then confirmed by a neuropsychiatrist, whose correct diagnosis led to significant improvement.

If both patient and physician are unaware that a concussion has occurred, many medical and neuropsychiatric problems may be misdiagnosed: Constant tiredness may be labeled chronic fatigue syndrome; depression may be misdiagnosed as manic-depressive disorder; those who complain of "hearing things" or "seeing things" may be called psychotic. People who seem overly concerned about their health may be dismissed as hypochondriacs. Seizures and migraine headaches may not be recognized as being part of post-concussion syndrome. Often the victims of post-concussion syndrome are called hysterics or malingerers (fakers), especially if a lawsuit is in progress; however, we have observed that in most of these situations, the symptoms continue even after the legal cases are settled.

Not everyone who has had a head injury develops post-concussion syndrome, but PCS should be suspected in anyone who has had a sudden altered mental state after a traumatic injury. A child who has had a concussion may have an unexplained personality change or may express a wish to stay home from school because of headaches or moodiness. The child's pediatrician should be told of any injuries from tripping and falling, being hit by a ball, or any other impact from contact sports or bicycle accidents prior to the onset of the new problems.

If you have a motor-vehicle accident that requires you to go to an emergency room, medical personnel usually focus their attention on visible injuries such as broken bones, cuts, and bruises. You may not be aware that you have had any loss of consciousness, and emergency-room staff usually do not question patients closely to find out whether a dysconscious episode occurred.

A useful questionnaire for a head-injured person would include, but not be limited to, the following questions:

- After an injury, have you felt confused, bewildered, dazed, or disoriented?
- Do you feel dizzy or light-headed?
- Do you feel physically off-balance? Do you stagger?
- Does it seem to you that time has slowed down, speeded up, or stopped? Do you feel that you have "lost" some time?
- Has your vision changed in any way? Are you experiencing a partial or complete loss of vision? Is your vision blurred or foggy? Do you see flashes of light, spots, or stars?
- Do you have double vision?
- Has your hearing changed? Do you hear bells or a ringing in your ears? Do sounds seem louder, muffled, distant, or strange?
- Are you in pain?

- Is any part of your body numb?
- Have you forgotten what happened right before your injury or just afterward? Do you have trouble remembering any recent or long-ago events?
- Do you feel anxious, depressed, panicky, paranoid, or angry?

If each of these symptoms is assigned a value of one point, the higher the score, the higher the probability of post-concussion syndrome. Using this system and saving the information could be very useful in predicting and treating future symptoms.

Any concussion makes its victim more vulnerable to any subsequent concussion. Some hidden concussions occur in patients who are already suffering from post-concussion syndrome. Patients and their doctors should be aware that any unexplained increase in headaches during the time of gradual recovery from an injury might be caused by minor head injuries overlooked by the patient and not reported to the doctor.

If you have had a concussion, you may misjudge distances. For example, you may bang your head on the door frame getting in and out of a car and think nothing of it. Something similar may happen at home and the incident may be overlooked. However, if you have had a minor head injury, a second minor head injury can cause persistent symptoms, slowing your recovery from your first injury. If you have had a recent injury, be sure to report any new injury to your physician, especially a head injury.

Many of us who have not had head injuries accidentally bang our heads on objects around the house such as a protruding cabinet or the top half of a Dutch door. However, a concussion can impair your overall judgment and awareness so that you forget the potential danger of protruding objects that you otherwise would avoid. Usually, your brain warns you of potential danger. But after a concussion, this awareness may be impaired, and the result may be multiple concussions. This can explain not only why you still hurt but also why you still keep getting hurt.

RECOGNIZING PCS

Post-concussion syndrome (PCS) may not be recognized until a patient is treated by a doctor or nurse who asks the right questions. Talk with your family physician if you experience any of these symptoms after an injury:

1. Headaches.
2. Nausea and vomiting.
3. Blurred vision.
4. Double vision.
5. Sensitivity to bright lights.
6. Impaired hearing.
7. Sensitivity to loud noises.
8. Ringing in the ears.
9. Dizziness.
10. Lightheadedness or blackouts.
11. Seizures.
12. Disorientation.
13. Balance problems.
14. Clumsiness or staggering.
15. Errors in depth perception.
16. Changes in handwriting.
17. Changes in color perception.
18. Changes in taste or smell.
19. Loss of appetite.
20. Increased appetite.
21. Junk food cravings.
22. Weight gain or loss.
23. Sleep disturbances.
24. Nightmares.
25. Daytime flashbacks.
26. Tiredness.
27. Irritability.
28. Difficulty concentrating.
29. Difficulty remembering recent events.
30. Difficulty finding words and expressing thoughts.
31. Difficulty following a sequence of directions.
32. Difficulty performing multiple tasks.
33. Difficulty understanding conversation.
34. Anxiety or fear, especially in an automobile.
35. Hallucinations.
36. Depression.
37. Menstrual changes.
38. Loss of ambition.
39. Loss of libido.
40. Loss of self-esteem.

Many of these individual symptoms can be attributed to other problems, such as post-traumatic stress and adjustment disorders. But when several of these symptoms occur together after a head injury, they form a picture of post-concussion syndrome. These symptoms are described in more detail below, and you'll find suggestions for treatment in Chapter 9.

UNDERSTANDING YOUR SYMPTOMS

The common symptoms of post-concussion syndrome include some or all of the conditions discussed in the section below.

Headaches

Headaches may be immediate or may not start until hours or even days after the impact. Ninety-five percent of patients who have had a concussion complain of headaches. Pain varies in its location, frequency, severity, and type. For the first few weeks, it may be constant and diffuse, throbbing or steady, sharp or dull. Sometimes it's more severe in the area of impact.

Some physicians make a distinction between headache and head pain. Head pain is more likely to be localized if the injury was caused by a blow or laceration. In cases of cervical sprain or strain (whiplash), the pain may start in the neck and radiate to the back of the head. If the back of your head was injured—for example, by forcefully hitting a headrest—a condition called "occipital neuropathy" may develop. In that event, the back of your head on one side or on both sides may be very tender to the touch and will require special treatment, which will be discussed in Chapter 9.

Sometimes, either direct injury to the jaws or forcible clenching of the jaws at the time of impact will injure the hinges of the lower jaw. Injured hinges are often tender to the touch, and the pain may be worse when biting or chewing. The pain may spread into the rest of the head.

Migraine headaches may begin after a concussion. Usually, this is because an old migraine problem is reactivated or aggravated by this injury. Migraine headaches may be accompanied by changes in vision, including shimmering effects or jagged, lightninglike flashes, numbness or weakness, or other strange feelings, usually preceding the head pain but sometimes occurring afterward or at the same time. The pain usually occurs on one side of the head and often causes nausea and vomiting. You probably will want to lie down in a dark, quiet room and sleep off a migraine.

You may not realize that you have had a concussion until you suddenly begin to have unrelenting headaches. Once you make the connection between your injury, your headaches, and other symptoms of post-concussion syndrome, you can discuss them with your physician so that proper studies can be done and the appropriate treatment started. Keeping a record of your headaches on a graph will help you and your doctor to observe the frequency of your headaches, your response to various medications, and your eventual gradual improvement.

If you are brought to an emergency room after an accident and a concussion is suspected, a CAT (computerized axial tomography) scan is usually recommended, especially if you complain of a headache or if other neurologic findings suggest a possible blood clot on the brain. Emergency-room staff usually give patients a "head sheet" with instructions for a responsible person to follow after release from the hospital. It would be helpful if emergency-room personnel also handed out information about the symptoms of post-concussion syndrome. This would tell patients what to expect and might lead to earlier treatment and a more speedy recovery with less of a psychological reaction.

Nausea and Vomiting

Nausea and vomiting usually occur within the first few days after a concussion, although nausea may persist for a longer period, gradually diminishing. Nausea and vomiting that occur at the scene of an accident warrant immediate, intensive medical attention to search for neurological causes of swelling in the brain.

Blurred Vision

Blurred vision very commonly occurs soon after a concussion. Usually, this clears up without treatment; however, post-concussion syndrome may hasten the need for reading glasses at an age earlier than you would otherwise expect.

Double Vision

Double vision is less common than blurred vision but is more serious. If it does not subside within a few weeks or if it remains constant from the outset, it is highly recommended that you see an ophthalmologist with neurologic training, because it may represent a serious injury.

Sensitivity to Bright Lights

Bright-light sensitivity may become a problem for the first time or may become more bothersome than it was before your injury. You may need to wear sunglasses outdoors more often and may want to turn down the lights when inside. While driving at night, you may be more sensitive to the headlights of oncoming vehicles.

Impaired Hearing

Impaired hearing may be the result of trauma to the ear, but it must be distinguished from difficulty interpreting what is heard. Being unable to understand conversation is a more frequent complaint than an actual loss of hearing.

Sensitivity to Loud Noises

Loud noises may become more annoying to you than they were before your injury. You may find yourself wanting to leave a theater before the movie is over because the sound system is overpowering. Crowds in which everyone is talking may be irritating, and you may even find less pleasure listening to music.

Ringing in the Ears (Tinnitus)

Tinnitus, or ringing in the ears, may be intermittent or constant. If it's intermittent, it usually improves. However, constant ringing is usually permanent and difficult to treat. Patients may also complain of other strange sounds (gurgling, rushing of water, chirping of crickets).

Dizziness

Dizziness, or a spinning sensation, is a common problem that may be caused by an injury to the balance mechanism in the ear (the labyrinth), especially if a blow has occurred on or near the ear. Sometimes dizziness is accompanied by headaches, nausea, and vomiting.

If episodes of dizziness do not decrease in frequency within a few weeks, consult an ear, nose, and throat specialist.

Lightheadedness

Lightheadedness is a common symptom and usually one of the first to subside, but it can continue for months. This faintlike feeling differs from dizziness because there is no spinning sensation. Like dizziness, it may be triggered by a sudden change in movement, especially if you get up too quickly from sitting or lying down. Lightheadedness may be severe enough to cause a blackout. However, a blackout (loss of consciousness) is not necessarily the same as a seizure. (See "Seizures" below.)

Seizures

Seizures are usually non-convulsive staring spells or "dropout" spells. These occur more frequently after a concussion than the older medical texts lead us to believe. In our experience with 6,000 cases, at least 5 percent of patients have had mild seizures intermittently.

Most seizures are staring spells, brief periods of staring with a gap in awareness. Dropout spells, which cause falling or dropping to the floor, are less frequent. Epileptic convulsions are rare. Any seizure that causes a change in conscious awareness should be reported to the state department of motor vehicles. Most states prohibit those who have had these spells from driving until they have been seizure-free for a specified period of time.

Disorientation

Episodes of disorientation may take place anywhere, including in your own home, in your car, or in your office. They may be very infrequent, or they may happen every day. They may last for a few seconds or a few minutes, and sometimes longer: Suddenly, you don't know where you are. This bewilderment creates anxiety. When you come out of it, you may find that you are in your car and that the road does not look familiar. Sometimes people pull off the road and wait until the feeling subsides. These episodes have been compared to minor seizures, but they have not yet been shown to cause any changes on an EEG.

Balance Problems

Problems with keeping your balance are usually temporary, unless your inner ear has suffered significant injury.

Clumsiness or Staggering

Clumsiness or staggering may, of course, be due to balance problems. Take extra care after a head injury to avoid climbing stepladders, bumping into door frames, and handling expensive china.

Errors in Depth Perception

Inability to perceive distances precisely may result in a partial loss of awareness of your surroundings. You may be surprised to find that you have bumped your head on a familiar door or archway when you were sure that you weren't anywhere near it.

Changes in Handwriting

Changes in handwriting may be so noticeable after a head injury that you may have to ask your bank to verify your new signature. However, you may be able to retain your identifying style if you concentrate and write slowly. Sometimes this symptom ultimately improves.

Changes in Color Perception

Changes in color perception may be subtle, such as not being able to tell the difference between navy blue and black. This is not the same as being color-blind (the inability to recognize certain colors from birth).

Changes in Taste or Smell

Changes in taste or smell are annoying and can even be dangerous if you lose the ability to smell smoke. This problem is often underdiagnosed because medical examiners do not routinely ask about it or test for it.

Loss of Appetite

Appetite loss may be caused by depression as a result of your head injury. If you become aware that you have lost your appetite, you may have to consciously encourage yourself to eat.

Increased Appetite

Increased appetite is a common problem that is somewhat more difficult to control than a loss of appetite. Knowing that this can be a symptom of post-concussion syndrome should encourage you to seek guidance from a nutritionist or your family physician.

Junk Food Cravings

Junk food cravings usually center on sweets or even on bizarre combinations of food like those pregnant women sometimes crave. People with post-concussion syndrome often crave chocolate and eat enormous amounts of it, even if they detested it before their head injuries.

Weight Gain or Loss

Weight gain or loss can result either from the concussion itself or from the medications used to counteract the anxiety or depression associated with post-concussion syndrome. Some people eat a lot when they are anxious; others eat less when they are depressed.

Sleep Disturbances

Sleep disturbances include difficulty falling asleep or staying asleep, or waking up too early in the morning. Whether caused by depression, anxiety, or physical changes that have taken place after a head injury, these problems can be treated in ways that are described in Chapter 9.

Nightmares

Nightmares may occur after a head injury, especially if the injured person also suffers from post-traumatic stress. This is an emotional problem caused by the frightening experience of an accident. However, nightmares also may be part of the post-concussion syndrome itself. Usually the nightmares are about accidents or some impending tragedy. These can be dealt with in therapy. Nightmares are discussed in Chapter 9.

Daytime Flashbacks

Like nightmares, daytime flashbacks are emotional reactions to an accident and are often triggered by seeing violence on television or by witnessing another accident. Merely hearing the screech of tires may be enough to create the recollection of your own accident.

It's been said that if you have been unconscious, there is no way that you could have a flashback of something you do not remember. Actually, some residual memory may exist, though it is repressed from your conscious memory.

Chronic Fatigue

Chronic fatigue after an injury is the result of injury to the brain, poor sleep patterns, and the extra mental energy needed to try to function normally. More energy is available in the morning, and some days are better than others. You should learn as quickly as possible when you have the most mental energy in order to know when to get important things done.

Irritability

Irritability can greatly interfere with your family relationships and your work. Rage reactions are not uncommon and, in some cases, have resulted in the loss of a job and the destruction of a marriage. Because rage reactions can be a form of seizures, a neurologist should be consulted.

Difficulty Concentrating

Concentration difficulties, one of the most common symptoms of post-concussion syndrome, is caused by impaired focusing. You may notice this symptom while you are watching television, or especially when you are trying to read a book or newspaper. Many post-concussion patients have temporarily given up reading. Those who have been able to continue to work have found that they have to reread things over and over again to grasp the meaning.

You may find it difficult to do two simple things at once, such as make breakfast while someone is talking to you. It may take a great deal of energy to focus on frying an egg. This problem also can cause you to make simple math errors when balancing your checkbook.

Short-Term Memory Problems

Short-term memory problems may be a significant part of post-concussion syndrome. You may leave the room to get something and forget what you wanted. You may forget appointments, birthdays, anniversaries, or telephone numbers. You may misplace objects and cash, or lock yourself out of the house or car. You may forget what has been said to others or what others have said to you.

Problems Verbalizing

Difficulty finding words and expressing thoughts (aphasia) can be annoying and embarrassing. After a head injury, you may have trouble remembering someone's name or finding a word you want to use in conversation; you may sometimes say the wrong word even though you know better. You might misquote what you are reading or have trouble reading aloud. You may begin to stutter for the first time, or, if stuttering was a problem years before, it may recur.

Difficulty Following a Sequence of Directions

Not being able to follow directions can be very frustrating. In the kitchen, you may have trouble following a recipe. At work, you may have similar problems following technical instructions. In the car, you may not be able to follow a map as easily as you did before your accident.

Difficulty Performing Multiple Tasks

Being unable to do more than one thing at a time may make your ordinary work more difficult. Doing more than one thing at a time can create such havoc that your efficiency drops considerably. Difficulty focusing and blocking out external distraction takes a great deal of energy, and you may tire more quickly than you would have before your head injury.

Difficulty Understanding Conversation

Difficulty understanding conversation is related to difficulty concentrating. This may be particularly troublesome when you are at a party where more than one conversation is going on at the same time. If the volume is too loud, it may override your ability to understand what is being said.

Anxiety

You may feel anxious or fearful in an automobile even if your head injury was not caused by a motor-vehicle accident. Your brain may seem to be more aware of the possibility of another concussion. This apprehension of potential risk sometimes reaches a level of paranoia, an unusual fear of vulnerability and a feeling that others are out to hurt you. You may not trust anyone's driving and may lose confidence in your own ability.

Hallucinations

Hallucinations that occur after a concussion are often so embarrassing that people do not mention them unless specifically questioned. Hallucinations are usually nothing more than hearing your name being called when there is no one there or hearing the telephone ring and there is no one on the line. Seeing "bugs" in your peripheral vision or even seeing things moving in the shadows is not uncommon. If this is happening, let your doctor know, and rest assured that it does not mean that you are going crazy.

Depression

Depression that is part of post-concussion syndrome has two main causes. The first is the physical injury to those areas of the brain that deal with emotions. The second cause is an emotional reaction to intellectual losses: You may feel that you have lost part of yourself, and you may go into partial mourning. Also, a preexisting manic-depressive disorder may be restarted or aggravated by a head injury.

Menstrual Changes

Changes in menstrual cycle can occur in any woman who has recently been through an emotionally disturbing experience, such as an accident. However, the brain's centers for hormonal regulation may have suffered microscopic damage from being jostled in the accident. Generally, these changes correct themselves.

Loss of Ambition

A loss of ambition can result from diminished mental and physical energy. You may find that you cannot think as efficiently as you used to and that you feel less creative. Some patients get involved in activities that they can no longer carry out and, in an effort to save face, quit trying.

Loss of Libido

A loss of libido is a common problem in people with PCS. The majority of these patients lose at least 50 percent of their sex drive, and others lose all of it. Certain medications, including some antidepressants, also may interfere with sexual responsiveness. It may take a long time to feel like yourself again, and it takes a great deal of understanding on the part of your sexual partner to maintain your relationship.

Loss of Self-Esteem

A loss of self-esteem can result from any of the symptoms of post-concussion syndrome: Each one interferes in its own way with your efficiency, your attention, and your interactions with others. This can make you feel less than who you once were.

Post-concussion syndrome can change your life so completely that you may feel and act like a different person. Unfortunately, you and your loved ones may not be fully aware of why you are no longer the same. Without proper treatment, marriages, friendships, and careers are at risk of being destroyed. Treatments for each of these symptoms, both traditional and alternative, are discussed in Chapter 9.

5

Complex Regional Pain Syndrome (CRPS) or Reflex Sympathetic Dystrophy (RSD)

SANJAY GUPTA, M.D.

More than 6 million people in the United States suffer from a painful condition called complex regional pain syndrome (CRPS), also known as reflex sympathetic dystrophy (RSD). This syndrome can become a devastating and incapacitating disease. The diagnosis is often missed or applied incorrectly to other conditions. It is very important that an accurate diagnosis be made as early as possible and that the syndrome be treated appropriately. Unfortunately, most of the time CRPS is diagnosed at an advanced stage, making treatment very difficult because of the significant damage that has occurred to the bones, blood vessels, and skin.

This condition was first described in 1864 by Civil War surgeons Mitchell, Morehouse, and Kane, who observed a series of typical changes in the hands and feet of wounded soldiers. Affected soldiers would fill their boots with water and wrap their injured limbs in rags to extinguish the "firelike" pain. The syndrome was originally named *causalgia* (in Greek, *causos* means "heat" and *algos* means "pain"), and people with CRPS typically do describe a "burning" type of pain. This pain can be greatly increased by sensations that are not normally painful, such as light pressure from sheets or clothes or even from air touching the skin.

For many years, the medical profession largely ignored this phenomenon or insisted that the pain was only in the patients' minds. The few physicians who did study this syndrome gave it many different names over the years, including causalgia, chronic traumatic edema, and shoulder-hand syndrome. It was not until 1993 that the International Classification of Disease (ICD) acknowledged RSD as a disorder. The following year, the International Association for the Study of Pain assigned this same disease the formal name complex regional pain syndrome (CRPS). Put simply, complex regional pain syndrome is the persistence of pain after any type of injury (or sometimes even without injury). The name itself, complex regional pain syndrome, reflects our incomplete understanding of this complex disorder. CRPS is usually localized to a specific region of the body; however, it has been known to spread to other parts of the body if left untreated. It is a dangerous myth that ignoring the pain and other symptoms will somehow make them disappear. In fact, delaying treatment will cause much more damage to develop.

Complex regional pain syndrome is classified into two types. Type I is known as RSD and type II is known as causalgia. The symptoms are similar or even identical in RSD and causalgia (see the chart on page 64); however, causalgia is diagnosed when an identifiable nerve injury exists.

CRPS affects three times more women than men. It occurs most frequently in the limbs, with the upper limbs more frequently affected than the lower limbs. Although this disorder usually affects only one side of the body, it occasionally occurs on both sides. It also can occur in other parts of the body, such as the neck, although this is less common.

The most common cause of CRPS is a fracture in the hand or leg; however, it can also result from any nerve or soft tissue damage. In addition to fractures, excessively tight application of casting materials, forceful manipulations, or surgical procedures may lead to CRPS. Some other common causes include sprains, dislocations, minor cuts, lacerations, contusions, crushing injuries, amputations, or gunshot wounds. Like carpal tunnel syndrome, CRPS can be caused by repetitive movements such as typing or machine operation. It is important to note again that it can happen after any minor or major injury or even without any identifiable injury. Approximately 33 percent of the cases of CRPS are without a known cause.

DIAGNOSTIC CRITERIA FOR CRPS TYPE I (RSD) AND CRPS TYPE II (CAUSALGIA)	
CRPS Type I or RSD	CRPS Type II or Causalgia
1) Continuation of pain, with a hypersensitivity to cold stimuli and nonpainful stimuli eliciting a pain response.	1) Continuation of pain, with a hypersensitivity to cold stimuli and nonpainful stimuli eliciting a pain response after a nerve injury, but not necessarily following the nerve distribution.
2) Evidence of swelling and skin changes with a decrease in blood flow to the affected area.	2) Evidence of swelling and skin changes with a decrease in blood flow to the affected area.
3) Absence of a condition that otherwise explains the above symptoms.	3) Absence of a condition that otherwise explains the above symptoms.
4) An inciting event or cause may or may not be present.	4) All three of the above must be present for this diagnosis.

The typical CRPS patient has a significantly painful cold, blue, sweaty limb. People often describe the pain as "burning" or "stabbing." The pain and appearance of the skin are usually worse when the limb is hanging down. If a person exhibits such symptoms as local skin-color changes and an excessive pain response to cold stimuli or light touch, it is likely that he or she is suffering from CRPS. Emotional distress, lack of sleep, and depression can also increase pain, as can loud noises or certain motions. The pain is also commonly worse at night.

STAGES OF CRPS

There are usually three stages of CRPS. It is important to note that the different stages may not follow the same chronological order in different individuals, and the presentation of particular symptoms can vary. In the first stage of CRPS, called the dysfunction stage, redness, swelling, and pain may be present. This stage usually lasts approximately three to six months. If treated in this stage, CRPS can be completely reversible.

If left untreated, CRPS will progress to the second stage, known as the dystrophy stage. A person in this phase exhibits cold and blue skin with sweating in a specific area, along with severe pain. The pain may become constant in this stage, and there may be signs indicating a loss of normal blood flow. Nails may become brittle, and bones may begin to show signs of osteoporosis or degeneration detectable by X-ray. This second stage lasts roughly six months, and CRPS is still reversible if treated during this period.

The third and final stage is atrophy (thinning or wasting of tissue). In this stage, there can be significant limb atrophy that results from both muscle and bone wasting. Eventually the limb becomes very painful and excessively atrophic. Joint contractures also may be present. In this late stage, the pain may start to subside; however, this does not signify that the CRPS is getting better. In fact, reduced pain at this point results from advanced tissue damage and is actually an ominous sign. It is very difficult for someone to recover if the disease has progressed to this stage.

WHY DOES CRPS OCCUR?

CRPS originated as a protective evolutionary mechanism, which can prove paradoxically harmful in our modern society. In the distant past, before the days of doctors and hospitals, if a person injured a limb, the body's first response was to send blood to that area to start the healing process. If the injury failed to heal after two to three weeks, the body's response was to shut down the blood supply to the limb, which was probably no longer useful. The limb turned cold and blue from the loss of blood flow. Most of this process, which causes the symptoms of CRPS, is most likely mediated by the sympathetic nervous system. This "fight-or-flight" system is responsible for constriction of blood vessels as well as other bodily functions. However, many experts believe that the sympathetic nervous system may be only partially responsible for the symptoms of CRPS or may be totally uninvolved in some cases. As you will later learn, an important aspect of the management of CRPS involves letting the brain know that the affected limb is still useful, so that the brain does not activate the sympathetic system and reduce the blood flow.

DIAGNOSING CRPS

The diagnosis of CRPS is usually based upon a physical exam, but there are some tests, such as a bone scan, that can be done to confirm the diagnosis. Evaluation of the bones will show changes similar to those in osteoporosis, because the bones degenerate from the lack of blood flow. However, bone findings vary greatly depending on the stage and progression of the disease: Even if the bone scan does not support the diagnosis, CRPS may still be present. Other tests such as the pseudo motor function test and thermography also may be used. Quantitative sensory testing (QST) is another test that is diagnostically useful, as it may detect CRPS in the earliest stages.

WHAT TO DO IF YOU SUSPECT CRPS

If you suspect you have CRPS, the most important thing to do is see your doctor immediately. If your doctor believes that you may have CRPS, he or she should initiate treatment or refer you to a board-certified pain specialist. The initial diagnosis is quite often missed, and the disease is allowed to progress because the person does not see a specialist in a timely manner. You can visit the Web site www.painguide.com for a list of pain centers that specialize in the management of CRPS. (Note that they may also use the term RSD.)

TREATMENT OF CRPS

Early treatment of CRPS is essential. The chances of recovery greatly improve with early detection and treatment. Sympathetic nervous system blocks are used for both diagnosis and treatment of CRPS. The sympathetic nervous system is the system that controls the closing and opening of the blood vessels. A physician who specializes in the treatment of CRPS can block this system with an injection, which can increase the blood flow to the area. This is done with the use of a local anesthetic, such as lidocaine, injected around the nerves to open the blood vessels to the limb. The injections are done in either the back or the neck, depending on which limb is affected. A catheter also can be inserted to provide a continuous infusion of this medication. Sometimes it is necessary to destroy the sympathetic nerves by surgical or chemical methods to improve the blood flow to the affected area.

There are many other treatment methods that should be used together for the best results. The most important and fundamental treatment is to make sure you still use the affected limb in some manner. As mentioned previously, it is very important to let the brain know that the limb is still useful. This can be done by simple techniques such as massage, paraffin wax, ultrasound, and physical rehabilitation. Your doctor can provide necessary pain medicine so you can continue to use the limb or do physical therapy to increase the blood flow. Some common medications used to treat CRPS and help control the pain are narcotic and non-narcotic analgesics, anticonvulsants, vasodilators, antidepressants, and antiarrhythmics. Some commonly used medications from these categories are Ultram, Darvocet, Daypro, Effexor, Neurontin, Gabatril, Zoloft, Clonidine, and Ketamine. The anti-inflammatory medications known as COX-2 inhibitors such as Vioxx and Celebrex can be very helpful in controlling the pain with fewer side effects. Local burning pain of CRPS sometimes responds very well to the use of a new transdermal patch called "Lidoderm patch." The patch uses the local anesthetic lidocaine to block the pain fibers in the skin. For intractable pain, stronger medications such as fentanyl can be given as a transdermal patch (Duragesic Patch) or orally (Actiq). If significant transdermal muscle spasm is present, a muscle relaxant such as Baclofen or the drug Zanaflex can be used.

Implantation of a spinal cord stimulator is a technique sometimes used in the management of CRPS. Small electrodes are placed via a minor surgical procedure into the spine; electrical stimulation then acts to mask the pain sensation and improve blood flow. By a similar principle, an external electrode device can be put on the skin to stimulate muscle fibers and skin, masking the pain. Two examples of such devices are a TENS unit and a sequential muscle stimulator (the latter is an advanced version of the TENS unit with additional useful features). If the pain is not controlled by these methods, a catheter (called an intrathecal pump) can be placed surgically into the spine to deliver pain medications directly into the spinal fluid.

Pain, especially in the form of complicated pain syndromes like CRPS, causes many psychological disturbances. For this reason, a behavioral or psychiatric consult is often useful to help you cope more effectively with the stress, emotional upset, or sleep problems that your pain may cause.

It is very important to have realistic expectations of the treatment process. The usual length of treatment is six months to a year, but it may take two or three years or even more if this disease is not caught until the advanced stages. Be patient, and continue your efforts during the entire length of the treatment.

One of the programs that we have found very useful in the treatment of CRPS is our mind/body program. In this program, we combine various alternative therapies with traditional treatments for the management of CRPS. We use several techniques, including biofeedback, acupuncture, hypnosis, massage therapy, aromatherapy, meditation, reflexology, and yoga, in order to gain better control over the pain of CRPS.

As emphasized earlier, if CRPS remains untreated, one can develop progressive pain and even limb loss. Here is an example of a patient we have successfully treated, in order to stress the point that CRPS can be well controlled if diagnosed and treated early. Our patient is a young woman in her twenties who fractured a small bone in the foot. She was in a cast for a few weeks and when the cast came off, she noticed that her foot was blue, cold, and painful. She went to her family doctor and was told that she really did not have any significant problem; she was instructed to wait and watch for improvement. She wisely sought a second opinion and was then referred to us at the Einstein Pain Center for treatment. We diagnosed her with CRPS and began treatment immediately. She underwent a sympathetic block as well as an infusion of local anesthetic in order to block both the sympathetic and peripheral nerves in her foot. Over the course of three to six months, her condition improved significantly.

Complex regional pain syndrome (CRPS) can be a painful and devastating condition that may lead to loss of the affected limb if not diagnosed early and treated properly. It is essential to consult a CRPS expert and begin a multi-modality treatment promptly. With early intervention, the chances of recovery are good.

HELPFUL WEB SITES AND ORGANIZATIONS

Amerian Pain Association
http://www.painassociation.org

Einstein Medical Center/Pain Center
5501 Old York Road
Willowcrest Bldg., 4th Floor
Philadelphia, PA 19141
Telephone: 215-456-PAIN

For support group infromation.

PainGuide
http://www.painguide.com

6

Mind/Body, Body/Mind, Mind/Brain, and Post-Traumatic Stress Disorder (PTSD)

JOSEPH C. NAPOLI, M.D.

"Which comes first—the chicken or the egg?" Ever since the accident, Sharon has been in a state of anxiety. Before the accident, she had felt in control of her life. At thirty-five years old, she had cared for her three children energetically and had worked part-time as a real estate salesperson. She and her husband had recently purchased their dream house. She was about to fulfill her goal of returning to school. Now she feels overwhelmed by the pain in her neck, back, and legs. She wonders how all this happened. What is causing this pain? she asks herself. Surely the injury to her skin, muscles, and other soft tissues was the source of this excruciating pain. But the accident had occurred months ago, and the swelling and bruises had subsided. Why is she still experiencing pain? When the pain occurs in the early morning, she blames her inactivity while sleeping for bringing it on. She attempts to work extra hard at her physical exercises to counteract her morning stiffness. Nevertheless, she is too exhausted to finish the regimen. When the pain begins later in the day, she attributes it to stress, especially because of her children's many needs. She feels guilty when she thinks, "If only I did not have the stress of so many responsibilities . . ." Then she thinks, " I'm not being a good mother when I wish that I did not have the responsibility of caring for my children. Maybe I deserve to be punished with this pain." Sharon's life has shrunk to being focused only on her pain. On her worst days, she loses her temper with her children or her husband. At the end of day, she sits alone weeping in the darkness. At the start of each new day, she attempts to grapple with the problem by asking herself, "What comes first? Does my pain cause my sadness and anger? Do my sadness and anger cause the pain? Do my anxiety and worry trigger the pain? I can't function with this pain, but if I don't work we won't have enough money and we'll lose the house. Why me? If I only knew where to start, I could . . ."

Post-traumatic pain can lead to a very vicious cycle from which one feels he or she cannot escape. Pain is a complex human experience. We divide to conquer. We separate out the parts in order to understand. Therefore, the solution to the puzzling problem of post-traumatic pain is to dissect pain into its parts. The hope for Sharon, and others like her who are lost in the dilemma of pain, is to look at the "trees" so that they can have the necessary knowledge of the "forest" that is needed to conquer the pain.

The anatomy (structure) that relates to pain is divided into the peripheral and central systems. The peripheral system consists of receptors (nociceptors [no-sih-SEP-turs]) in the skin, muscles, internal organs, and other tissue that perceive noxious, or physically harmful, stimuli and "wires" (peripheral nerves) that connect these receptors to the "main transmission cable" (the spinal cord). The spinal cord is connected to the brain by way of the brain stem. The spinal cord and the brain comprise the central system (the central nervous system). However, this brief description of the "hardwiring" does not explain the components of the pain experience. In other words, how does this structure function?

A simple model of the pain experience would be that a noxious stimulus causes activation of specific pain sensors, which results in the one-way transmission of a signal from the sensor to a "pain center" in the brain. For example, with regard to post-traumatic pain, the stimulus might be a blow to the body. In this view of pain, the brain functions merely as a passive organ that registers the pain sensation. The intensity of the pain is proportional to the intensity of the stimulus—the greater the blow, the greater the pain. This model of pain, called the *specificity theory,* is a legacy of the philosopher René Descartes who put forth his explanation of pain c. 1633. Ironically, the man whose philosophy was "I think, therefore I am" did not think there was any role for "thought" in the pain experience. Because physicians were straddled with this "mindless" understanding of pain for three centuries, there was no appreciation of an active role for emotion and thought in the pain experience. Scientists thought that emotion related to pain only as a secondary reaction of the pain sufferer.

This limited view of pain began to change in 1965 when Patrick D. Wall and Ronald Melzack proposed the *gate control theory of pain.* They postulated that 1) signals are transmitted in two directions—nerve impulses travel from the receptors to the brain, and modulating nerve impulses travel from the brain in the opposite direction, and 2) neural "gate" mechanisms in the spinal cord open and close in order to allow or stop the traveling of nerve impulses. This theory clearly emphasizes the key role of the central nervous system. Subsequently, Melzack elaborated on the function of the brain by formulating three components of the pain experience—the *sensory-discriminative,* the *cognitive-evaluative,* and the *emotional-motivational.* Although the gate control theory does not accommodate all of the scientific data that has been collected about pain, it has been very useful in clarifying the role of the mind/brain in the pain experience, especially when the pain is chronic. Shortly, I will present aspects of the mind/body interaction and the mind/brain integration and how these relate to the experience and control of post-traumatic pain.

In addition to these general aspects of the mind/brain that can be applied to the understanding of post-traumatic pain, there is a specific mental disorder—post-traumatic stress disorder (PTSD)—that develops after an individual has been exposed to a traumatic event and that can complicate the post-traumatic pain experience. Whereas post-traumatic pain originates from a direct injury, PTSD is a psychologically mediated disorder with biological components. In other words, the seeing, hearing, and smelling of a traumatic event, along with our emotional and cognitive responses to the trauma, can cause biological reactions in our brains. These biological reactions may persist and develop into PTSD. Both the intensity of the event and individual predisposition play a role in the development of this disorder. Thus, PTSD is a condition in which the mind (the psychological) produces changes in the brain, and these brain (the biological) changes affect the mind. Although PTSD and post-traumatic pain are separate entities, it is useful to consider them together because when they both result from the same trauma, they can adversely impact each other. Therefore, after reviewing the general aspects of mind/brain/body in regard to pain, I will focus on PTSD as a disorder that often may accompany post-traumatic pain and as a model that illustrates the general aspects of the role of mind/brain in the pain experience.

MIND/BODY

"Pain, no gain." The burn-unit surgeons and nurses were frustrated and very concerned. Sixteen-year-old Juan was refusing to participate in the physical therapy that was essential for his rehabilitation. The staff thought that surely he must be depressed or have some personality disorder. How else could one explain his behavior that was nullifying all the operations he had undergone for his extensive second- and third-degree burns? The most difficult part of the treatment had been completed, but without Juan's active participation in his recovery, he would develop skin deformities and muscle wasting. Juan would never walk again. When I saw him for a psychiatric consultation, he confessed what he was too ashamed to tell the other doctors, especially because they were trying to encourage him with the motto "No pain, no gain." He had a reputation in his neighborhood of being a tough kid, but now he had to admit that he wept frequently because he could not tolerate the pain. He had decided that the "brave" thing to do was to accept being an invalid. Fortunately, Juan proved to be hypnotizable. Therefore, he was able to learn self-hypnosis and use it to master his pain. The staff thought that it was a miracle when Juan began to walk without any pain and with a proud smile. With hypnosis, Juan achieved a tremendous gain without any pain.

What is this process we call hypnosis that has engendered so many myths? It is *not* being under the spell of someone else who tells you to cluck like a chicken. It is *not* being in a state of sleep, contrary to the Greek meaning of the word—(*hypnos*, meaning "sleep") and (*osis,* meaning "condition"). It is *not* a sure path to the truth. It is *not* even powerful. The power is in our minds. Hypnosis is only a tool to tap into this power. What is this power of the mind? How does hypnosis help us use it to master pain?

Attention is the mental activity that is the power of the mind. There are some well-known examples of how attention, or its opposite—distraction—can make us oblivious to pain. "Battlefield analgesia," which was observed during World War II, occurs when a soldier, although seriously wounded, feels no pain while he is still on the battlefield focusing on the danger around him. When he is safely evacuated to the field hospital, he experiences intense pain because he is no longer distracted by the bullets and mortars that were threatening his life. A civilian example of this type of "painkiller" is the athlete who is injured but keeps playing without any sense of pain because he or she is focused on winning the game. Feats of superhuman strength—like a mother who saves her child's life by lifting heavy debris that is trapping him—also demonstrate this power of the mind.

The state of hypnosis has two elements: 1) focused attention by altered consciousness, and 2) heightened suggestibility. Hypnosis augments the human capacity to focus attention by means of altered consciousness. *Dissociation* is a mechanism of the mind that separates the usually integrated functions of the mind. Thoughts, memories, perceptions, and emotions are separated from conscious awareness or from one another by the process of dissociation. Some people can go into a trance and not be consciously aware of their surroundings. For example, as I am sitting at my computer, I can be so highly focused on writing this paragraph that I am oblivious to the passage of time and to someone calling me. Individuals have a greater or lesser degree of this capacity to dissociate and enter a state of altered consciousness. The hypnotist facilitates a person's entering into a trance, that is, a dissociative state. Hence, hypnosis achieves a heightened state of awareness by paradoxically limiting awareness. Therefore, hypnosis allows one to use the power of attention in a very magnified way so that it excludes all other stimuli. In a state of hypnosis, one is very suggestible. During the trance state, the perception of pain can be blocked. In addition, those people who are very hypnotizable experience post-trance amnesia; that is, they do not remember having undergone the hypnosis, and are influenced by posthypnotic suggestion. For example, when these people are in a hypnotic state and are told that they will feel no pain after they are out of the trance, they do not experience any pain even when they are no longer in the hypnotic state. Therefore, hypnosis can be used as a tool to control pain while either in the trance state or in the posthypnotic state. Regrettably, although the phenomenon of hypnosis has been used within the field of medicine since the eighteenth century, it is still greatly underutilized for pain control, especially in dental and surgical procedures, except for the Lamaze childbirth method. This underutilization is based largely on the perception of hypnosis being some sort of magic trick without scientific merit. Nevertheless, there are data about the biology of hypnosis. For example, PET scans (an imaging technique that shows blood flow activity) of the human brain during pain stimuli demonstrate activity in an area called the anterior cingulate cortex. This brain area is also central to the function of attention. Interestingly, in another study, when a person was given a hypnotic suggestion to reduce the unpleasantness of a noxious pain stimulus, the activity in the anterior cingulate cortex was reduced.

How else might we use this power of our minds? Common sense, like the lyrics of the Johnny Mercer song, tells us that "You got to ac-cent-tchu-ate the positive / e-lim-i-nate the negative / and latch on to the affirmative . . ." Although we should use the power of our minds to think positively, unfortunately, we human beings are champions at focusing on the negative. Complaints, gripes, and criticisms are in abundance. It is easy to be a Monday morning quarterback. We tend to better register the slights, remember the bad times, and dwell on the hurtful remarks. Maybe from the standpoint of individual self-protection this is adaptive behavior. Maybe accentuating the negative is "hardwired" in our brains because it has provided us with an advantage in the evolutionary struggle to survive. For example, perhaps the younger members of the tribe learned about the dangers out on the savannah because Og repeatedly related his "war story" to his fellow cavemen sitting around the fire about the terrible, tragic hunt when a saber-toothed tiger devoured Lug.

The negative is automatic; we have to work at the positive. Corporations, health-care facilities, and service organizations overwhelm us with "satisfaction surveys." Complaints will always come uninvited; praise has to be harvested. My unsolicited gripe is that I am fed up with being asked to fill out so many satisfaction surveys! Nevertheless, J. D. Power's thriving survey business is a sign that these questionnaires are completed and that there is a need to measure the positive as well as the negative views. Norman Vincent Peale's *The Power of Positive Thinking,* the granddaddy of self-help books, was an international best-seller because its inspirational message helped to fill the void of insufficient positive thinking. Likewise, present-day self-help and guidance books such as this one fill the need that we have to be either taught or reminded and coached about positive thinking. Thus, we should use the power of our minds—

attention—to key in on positive thoughts. Our minds can consciously concentrate on only one thought at a time. On the one hand, by telling ourselves not to think negatively, we are concentrating on the negative. On the other hand, if we train our minds on a positive thought, this action blocks out negative thoughts. Positive thoughts can be structured in the form of an affirmation—for example, "I am in control." Because hypnosis is focused attention and suggestion, an affirmation is reinforced when stated or heard in a hypnotic trance. Thus, hypnosis can aid our positive thinking.

Like expert opinion on so many things, there are at least two schools of opposing opinion regarding the capacity to be hypnotized. The opinion of Milton Erickson that anyone can be hypnotized is at odds with the position of Herbert Spiegel that not all people can be hypnotized. According to Spiegel, hypnotizability, that is, the ability to be hypnotized, is an inborn capacity. Some are completely without this capacity. Those who have the capacity have it to varying degrees. On one end of the spectrum are people with low hypnotizability and on the other end are people with high hypnotizability.

I was trained by Dr. Spiegel, and the data in my clinical practice regarding hypnotizability support his opinion. This might be disappointing news to you, especially if, as you read this book, you were thinking that, like Juan, you might be miraculously "cured." Do not give up hope. First, you might be highly hypnotizable. (See "Dr. Herbert Spiegel's Eye-Roll Test," Figure 6.1 on page 77.) Second, motivation is a key aspect for the use of hypnosis. I have seen people who fight against going into a trance although they have an inborn capacity to be hypnotized. I have seen other people so highly motivated that with practicing self-hypnosis they achieve benefit even though they have low hypnotizability. Third, there are other methods that one might use to focus their attention on mastering their post-traumatic pain. These methods are relaxation, biofeedback, and imagery.

"Just relax" is often frustrating advice for the post-traumatic pain patient. The pain sufferer usually replies, "If I could so easily relax, I would have already done it." or "This ____ pain doesn't let me relax." (You fill in the blank.) Once you know that the mind influences the body, relaxing is actually an excellent idea. But a person, especially one suffering with pain, cannot "just relax." They need to learn a relaxation technique, practice the technique, and become skilled at doing it.

Dr. Herbert Spiegel's Eye-Roll Test

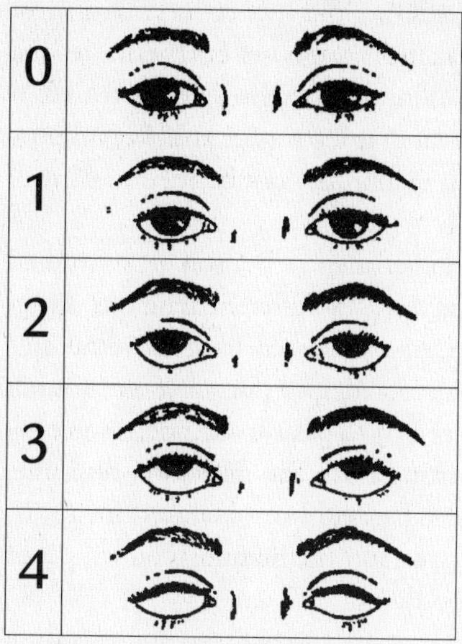

0 = not hypnotizable
1 = low hypnotizability
2–3 = midrange of hypnotizability
4 = high hypnotizability

Ask someone to observe your eyes while you perform the steps below. He/she should rate from 0 to 4 how much of the white portion of your eyes is showing during Step 3 by comparing your eyes to the chart at the left.

Step 1. ***Keeping Head Still*** Hold your head straight and look forward.

Step 2. ***Upward Gaze*** As you hold your head in this position, look upward toward the top of your head.

Step 3. ***Eye-Roll*** As you continue to look all the way upward, slowly close your eyelids.

Step 4. ***Return to the Usual Focus*** Open your eyelids and let your eyes come back into focus.

This is a quick screening method to test hypnotizability. It was developed and studied by Herbert Spiegel, M.D. 73.9% of persons who are rated as hypnotizable on this eye-roll test are able to enter a hypnotic state when they have undergone a full hypnotic induction. If you have a good eye-roll and would like to use hypnosis for pain control and/or relaxation, please inform your physician. You should only use hypnosis under the guidance of an appropriately trained health-care professional.

FIGURE 6.1

Beginning in 1968, Herbert Benson, M.D., a cardiologist who was concerned about hypertension and the effects of stress on the cardiovascular system, studied the physiological effects of transcendental meditation (TM). He and his colleagues discovered that meditation elicits an innate human capacity that counteracts stress. He called this capacity the relaxation response. Contrary to the human stress response, the relaxation response decreases oxygen consumption, respiratory rate, heart rate, and blood pressure. When the electrical activity of the brain is measured by an electroencephalogram (EEG), alpha waves increase in frequency and intensity during the relaxation response. Furthermore, the levels of lactate, a chemical product of muscle activity, are decreased. It has been repeatedly demonstrated in laboratory studies that lactate produces panic attacks. Hence, relaxation techniques can be used to control panic attacks.

Fascinated by the results of his experiments, Benson next studied prayer and meditation as they are practiced by different religions. From these prayer and meditation methods, he extracted four universal elements—1) a quiet environment, 2) a mental device (focusing on a sound, word, or phrase, or gazing on an object), 3) a passive attitude, 4) a comfortable position—that combine to bring forth the relaxation response. Thus, this scientific work reaffirmed what had been believed for thousands of years in religion, that is, prayer and meditation produce peace and harmony within the mind and body.

Biofeedback is a method of training oneself to achieve the relaxation response by having a machine measure certain biological parameters—brain waves, blood pressure, heart rate, muscle tension, and skin temperature—of the relaxation response. While hooked up to a measuring device, the patient learns to control these usually involuntary functions by relaxing while the machine informs the patient—that is, feeds back information about these parameters—that he or she is achieving control.

Imagery is focusing on pictures in your mind. For example, one can think of pleasant pictures such as being in a peaceful place. Athletes use imagery in their training to improve their performance. For example, when runners visualize themselves in motion, muscles are actually activated as measured with a machine called an electromyograph. Thus, they develop a "muscle memory" for the action of running. A laboratory study that used the cold-pressor pain test (a person's limb is placed in very cold water) demonstrated that imagery training increased the threshold of experiencing the pain. Imagery can be combined with relaxation techniques or hypnosis.

There is a risk in our placing all our expectations for the mastery of pain in the power of the mind and in the "mind over body" point of view. When a person does not sufficiently benefit from these mind methods—hypnosis, positive thinking, relaxation, biofeedback, and imagery—he or she might blame himself or herself. "If only I had done the method correctly it would have worked. It would have relieved my pain" is a common but not necessarily correct refrain. The fact that this is negative thinking "rearing its ugly head" is not missed by the patient, who continues, "There I go again, dwelling on the negative. I'm so self-defeating." This self-blame may not be justified. First, no method is 100-percent effective 100 percent of the time. Therefore, the method may have failed you; you may not have failed at using the method. Second, as I explain in this chapter, pain, especially chronic post-traumatic pain, is a very complex phenomenon with multiple components. Therefore, the mind over body method is only one tool of a multi-modality approach to post-traumatic pain management. Third, negative thinking and pain are both powerful phenomena that we are unable to just will away. Persistence and efforts that are supported by health professionals, family, and friends—and for many patients, self-help groups—are essential to mastering pain.

BODY/MIND

"I'll never be the same." It was a terrible industrial accident. Ann's hand was caught and crushed. Although the surgeons tried to save it, amputation became necessary. It wasn't just the phantom pain (a feeling that her painful hand was still present) that was troubling her. She could not accept the loss of her hand. She felt different. She felt like a freak. Various well-meaning family members and friends tried to cheer her up and help her get over it. Nevertheless, her sadness increased with each platitude that she heard, including, "It is only your left hand and you are right-handed." "It could have been worse." "You shouldn't be feeling any pain; your hand is not there." "Look at it this way, there are people without any legs." "You should be happy that you still have your right hand and that you can work." As the days continued, her grieving worsened, and she cried every day, lost her appetite, developed insomnia, lost interest in her hobbies, withdrew from socializing, was unable to concentrate, and began to plan her suicide. She felt worthless without her hand and guilty that she was not "strong enough" to bear the physical pain.

Ann is an example of a person who develops a psychiatric disorder after suffering a traumatic injury to her body. Our minds do react to what occurs in our bodies. We think, feel, and behave in response to experiencing pain. However, there is no direct biological link between Ann's bodily pain and the reaction of her brain in developing the psychiatric disorder. As human beings, we react psychologically to pain and loss. We not only weep for a loved one who has died but also feel sorrow for strangers when we hear that they have perished. As a nation, we grieved for those who died in the terrorist attacks on September 11, 2001. We lament the painful suffering of others. Therefore, the bond is psychosocial and not biological. Although Ann's loss is not the death of another but the loss of part of her body, her grief is psychologically connected to her loss. Likewise, other trauma survivors may react emotionally to the loss caused by their chronic post-traumatic pain—such as loss of function and loss of quality of life. When psychiatric disorders are triggered in this way, we call them "reactive" or "secondary."

Some people may not be surprised that Ann became depressed after such a tremendous loss. However, they might consider it a normal reaction to a horrible injury and thus not appreciate that she is experiencing clinical depression that requires treatment. Undergoing a stressor such as post-traumatic pain, on the one hand, may generate normal anxiety and sadness; on the other hand, it may produce anxiety and depressive disorders. It is important to recognize and get treatment for these disorders because such disorders intensify pain and are associated with the risks of 1) self-medication with alcohol and drugs and 2) suicide.

Unlike "reactive" or "secondary" disorders, there are phenomena that occur in our bodies that have a direct biological influence on our thoughts, emotions, and well-being. We can actually "muscle" our brains—have a biological impact on our moods and pain experience—by the activity of our bodies. In contrast to the mind activity of hypnosis and meditation, neuromuscular relaxation is a technique that focuses on the body. The experiments of E. Gellhorn demonstrated that feedback from the skeletal muscles affects the hypothalamus, a part of the brain that is central to the control of the stress response and the relaxation response. Therefore, when a patient progressively tenses (contracts) and relaxes selected muscles under the guidance of a therapist, a relaxation response occurs and the patient's anxiety subsides. Likewise, rigorous exercise has an impact on the chemistry of our brains. Exercise stimulates the production of brain endorphins—the brain's natural painkillers. Regular exercise is an essential component to recovering from post-traumatic pain. The activity of the body has a healthy effect on the mind that, in turn, heals the body. Thus, this interaction restores a "healthy mind in a healthy body."

There are popular phrases about emotion that are metaphorically related to the "gut," that is, the stomach and the intestines—anxiety ("I have butterflies in my stomach"), emotional hurt ("That remark hit me right in the gut"), fear ("I was shitting in my pants"), and anger ("My stomach is growling"). Why do we use digestive system metaphors to express our emotions? Is this a body/mind connection? Is this another example of how the biological mechanisms in our bodies affect the emotions of our minds? Is there a feedback mechanism from the "gut" to the brain? In his book *The Second Brain,* Michael Gershon explains that "gut instinct" may have to do with the serotonin (a neurotransmitter) produced in the gut. This enteric serotonin is the same as the serotonin secreted in the brain that is involved in many psychobiological mechanisms including those for anxiety, depression, and pain. Therefore, by the fact that serotonin is produced in the gut, our bowels may have a direct influence on our emotions, behavior, and pain experience. Although medications that might act specifically on the serotonin system in the gut are being researched, it is too early to know if another way to control pain may be through our stomachs.

A cascade of chemicals—including bradykinin, leukotrienes, nerve growth factor, prostaglandins, serotonin, and substance P—activates in response to trauma to the body and is part of the immediate inflammatory process. Although these chemicals are a rapid response "team" that protects our bodies, they also intensify the perception of pain. This could be another way the body affects the mind/brain. Acute trauma might initiate an "imprint" or "memory" of pain in the central nervous system that under certain conditions persists after the acute pain and inflammation subside. Quick and thorough pain relief is crucial to acute pain management. It is assumed that by mitigating the intensity and duration of the pain, it is less likely to form an "imprint." Medications are primary interventions in acute pain management. NSAIDs (nonsteroidal anti-inflammatory drugs)—for example, aspirin and ibuprophen—interfere with prostaglandin production. Opioids—for example, codeine, morphine, and oxycodone—reduce neurotransmitter (nerve chemical) release or nerve sensitivity.

MIND/BRAIN

"When it rains, I feel pain." Margaret, a sixty-three-year-old widow, easily tells the story of that fateful day. While driving her car, she was rounding that curve as she had done often in the past. This time, her car slid into a harrowing skid on the wet autumn leaves scattered on the road. She recalls the police officer covering her head and shoulders with a blanket to protect her from the drizzling rain. Although her car crashed down an embankment, she felt lucky that she sustained no head injury or broken bones. Furthermore, she thought she had no psychological effects from the accident. Her only suffering was "this damn aggravating pain in my neck and back" that was ruining her life. Some days it was hardly noticeable; other days it became terribly intense. It was very puzzling until her friend asked, "Have you ever noticed that your pain acts up on rainy days?" And Margaret replied, "I never noticed that. But you are right. When it rains, I feel pain." After her friend's comment, Margaret also admitted that she had stopped leaving her home because her pain was more intense if she ventured out. She began by staying at home only on rainy days. Eventually, she never left at all.

Although Margaret described her rainy painful days as "days not fit for a dog," she did not know that it is Pavlov's dog experiments that explain the connection between her pain and the rain. A dog's natural response is to salivate when given food. This well-known physiologist discovered that by ringing a bell when he presented food to a dog, the dog eventually "learned" to salivate when only the bell was rung. Classical conditioning or learning consists of an unconditioned stimulus (for example, food or Margaret's accident) being paired with a conditioned stimulus (the bell or the rain). Initially, only the unconditioned stimulus produces a response (the dog's salivating or Margaret's pain). Later, the conditioned stimulus alone produces this same response.

Margaret was also unaware that her behavior of avoidance (shutting herself in her home) actually worsened her pain. How could this be? Her common sense told her the exact opposite, that is, her pain lessened when she avoided going out, and intensified when she left her home. However, we know from the research originally of Edward L. Thorndike on trial-and-error learning and then of B. F. Skinner that behavior which is rewarded is reinforced. Initially, Margaret went out when it rained and her pain intensified (aversive stimulus). However, when she retreated back to her home (a response to the aversive stimulus), her pain lessened (a reinforcer or reward for her behavior). Thus, she learned to escape her pain (escape learning). This is the beginning of the downward spiral experienced by people with chronic pain.

Next, Margaret anticipated that if she went out she would be inflicted with intense pain (aversive stimulus). She feared that she would experience pain. Hence, she avoided going out (anticipatory response) and did not experience the aversive stimulus (avoidance learning). Her pain not becoming more intense is a reinforcer for her not to leave her home. It also reinforces her fear of experiencing pain and leads to ever decreasing activity. By being isolated at home, she engages in less physical activity and restricts her socializing. She is no longer distracted by engaging in outdoor activity while accompanied by her friends. Without sufficient physical activity, her pain worsens. Without social involvement, she feels alone and sad. Without distractions, her thoughts are fully focused on her pain. As her pain worsens, so does her anxiety. Her attention to her pain, anxiety, and depression aggravates her pain. Her agony becomes worse. Her quality of life spirals further and further downward.

A more common and less drastic example of this avoidance learning in patients with post-traumatic pain occurs when they do not engage in physical therapy. Although by avoiding physical therapy they do not experience an aggravation of their pain during and in the aftermath of the physical therapy, without the physical therapy the body stiffens and the pain progressively becomes worse.

The psychotherapy solution for Margaret's pain was her being armed with this knowledge about the conditioned aspect of her pain, and her deliberately going forth even on rainy days. This behavior progressively desensitized her brain, that is, broke the unconscious link between her pain and the rain. Therefore, rainy days no longer triggered her pain. In addition, she used conditioning to change her behavior by rewarding herself—going to a favorite place, dining with a special friend, or shopping for a gift for herself—whenever she forced herself to leave her home. By deliberate effort that we planned together, she was able to shape her behavior and master her pain instead of unconsciously and automatically reacting to triggers of her pain.

You might be thinking that this was fine for Margaret who had a simple trigger for her pain. Further, you might be thinking, "No matter what I do I suffer with pain. If I go out, I experience pain. If I stay home,

I experience pain. If I sit, I experience pain. If I stand, I . . . etc., etc., etc. No matter what, I feel totally helpless. I have no control over anything." If this describes you, then you are caught in a state of learned helplessness. In order to help yourself, you should consider the work of Martin Seligman, who developed the learned helplessness model based on his "inescapable shock" animal studies. First, he and his colleagues placed the test animal in a hammock that prevented it from escaping from an aversive but physically harmless stimulus that was applied to the animal. Second, they placed this animal in a box from which it could easily escape a shock by moving into another compartment of the box. When an aversive stimulus was applied, the animal did react to it but then became very passive and did not move into the other compartment to escape the shock. Third, when they placed another test animal, which had never received inescapable shocks in a hammock, in the box and applied the aversive stimulus, this animal moved and escaped the shock. Therefore, they taught an animal to be helpless. Pain teaches the pain sufferer to be helpless. Helplessness is a psychological state in which events are perceived to be uncontrollable. No matter what you do, it does not matter. What you do does not change anything. There is no way out, or so you think.

Thinking makes it so. People are not actually helpless unless they think they are. If you think you are helpless, you will not be motivated and will not initiate any action to take control and change a situation. Human subjects in a laboratory study who believed that they were controlling the duration of a painful stimulus experienced less pain and withstood higher levels of pain compared with subjects who believed that they had no control over how long the pain stimulus was applied. The person with chronic pain develops a repertoire of self-defeating pain behaviors that are all part of learned helplessness. It is difficult to change this negative thinking because learned helplessness interferes with learning. In the face of apparently uncontrollable pain, the pain sufferer has difficulty recognizing that his or her attempts to ameliorate the pain have been successful. The post-traumatic pain sufferer should behave similarly to the mother who responds, "Have you tried it?" to her child who says, "I don't like that food." Instead of putting off an idea (no matter who originates it) that might benefit him or her with the excuse—"It will never work"—the post-traumatic pain sufferer should ask him- or herself, "Have I tried it?" Also, trying a methodology once is most likely not enough. It usually has to be done repeatedly in order for it to be successful. Seligman got his animals out of their state of learned helplessness by repeatedly picking them up and moving them into the other compartment of the box, away from the shock. He needed to actually move the animals because learned helplessness interferes with one's motivation to initiate voluntary responses to control events. Therefore, when the pain sufferer feels helpless, he or she should try something anyway or allow someone to figuratively pick him or her up by "the scuff of the neck" and place him or her in a different setting. Firmly encouraging the learned helplessness pain patient to partake in activity is an important role for family and friends. Furthermore, by participating in the activity with the pain sufferer, family and friends provide support and reward for the person's not engaging in his or her pain behavior.

Cognitive appraisal is a mental process of interpreting the world as it unfolds before a person. We assign meaning to what happens around and to us. Therefore, what happens is in the "eye of the beholder." One person's pain is another person's challenge. Thus, the meaning that we apply to our pain influences the chronic pain experience. Negative meanings, such as Sharon's thinking that her pain is punishment for her guilt, might intensify the pain, whereas a positive meaning, such as "pain will make me tough," might make it more tolerable. How we appraise things in the present is based on cognitive perceptions or beliefs that developed in our past, especially in our childhood.

Another mental activity is *attribution*—the process by which we assign motive to our behavior or someone else's behavior. Answers to "Why me?" can be attributions. For example, a person may blame himself for causing the accident that injured him. Self-blame is not necessarily a bad thing. Taking responsibility for one's actions provides one with a sense of control and may lead to a change in behavior that produces a better outcome. For example, a person thinks, "This time, I made a mistake. Next time, I will know how to protect myself." This is behavioral self-blame. A person who thinks "I never do anything right" is engaging in characterological self-blame. This is very self-defeating. If you have such an attitude of ineffectiveness, it only places you at the mercy of your pain and increases your suffering. Self-efficacy—the belief in one's effectiveness—is important for coping with pain.

What we think affects how we feel and behave. This idea is central to the cognitive theory developed by Aaron Beck in 1969. Thus, our cognitive appraisals and attributions influence our emotions. You might automatically think, "People will laugh at me if I walk with a cane." You might automatically think, "If I venture outside, I will be injured again." These "automatic thoughts" or "cognitive distortions" will prevent you from being active. Automatic thoughts are the result of underlying maladaptive assumptions, that is, patterns of thinking. "Cognitive errors" result from these assumptions. For example, the cognitive error called "catastrophizing" results from the assumption that "the worst will always happen to me." Studies have demonstrated that catastrophizing is related to greater pain intensity, more impairment, and/or worse treatment outcome. In addition, pain sufferers have a heightened awareness of pain-related stimuli (attentional bias). The hope for people who demonstrate cognitive errors and attentional bias is cognitive therapy that can be used to change how we think. Through the process of cognitive therapy, a person can learn to recognize his or her automatic thoughts, identify the underlying maladaptive assumptions, and correct the thinking that has led to anxiety, depression and/or the worsening of his or her pain and suffering.

What role do our emotions play in the experience of pain? Although it is debatable whether emotions cause pain, they certainly can aggravate pain. Anxiety, with its worry and muscle tension, makes pain more intense. Anger, either suppressed or ragefully released, increases the stress in our systems and intensifies pain. It is intriguing to note that the Latin verb *dolère* means both "to feel pain" and "to grieve." The ancient Romans apparently believed that there is a close association between physical pain and the emotional pain of mourning. I have seen many grieving patients who describe their anguish in bodily terms. Recently, I treated a man whose sibling had died in the World Trade Center terrorist attack. He recalled that when he heard the news, he let out a cry and felt an intense wave of physical pain travel from his head to his feet. Part of mastering post-traumatic pain is working through your feelings, especially about the traumatic event and its consequences.

For many years, medical science rested on the assumption that our brains do not change except for losing cells and function during the course of our lives. Now we believe in brain plasticity, that is, the ability of the brain to be flexible and change in response to stimuli. Since the brain is composed of chemicals, the idea that chemical agents can change the brain is accepted as reality. Antidepressant medication relieves depression. L-Dopa reduces the symptoms of Parkinson's disease. Alcohol, nicotine, and other drugs affect the brain. But is the environment able to change our brains? Do our behaviors change our brains? Does psychotherapy alter the biology of the brain? The answer to all these questions is "yes." The seminal work of psychiatrist and Nobel laureate Eric Kandel has demonstrated the plasticity of the cell neuron of the *Aplysia,* a sea snail, in regard to the functions of learning and memory. In addition, a brain imaging study demonstrated that London cab drivers have a significantly larger volume of the area of the brain essential for factual memory called the hippocampus. Thus the environmental demand of needing to learn and remember the streets of London produced a change in their brains. A 1992 brain imaging study of patients with obsessive-compulsive disorder (OCD) demonstrated that behavior therapy produced blood flow changes in the same area of the brain as medication treatment. There are "maps" or representations of our bodies in our brains. Brain imaging has demonstrated that right-handed violinists have a larger map of their left hands, which perform all the intricate fingering of the violin strings, compared with their right hands, which merely move the bow back and forth. In one study, a person who had lost both hands in an accident had a decreased map upon brain imaging in reference to his missing hands. After the person underwent hand transplant surgery, the hand representation in the brain expanded to recognize the transplanted hands.

These studies demonstrate that our brains change through psychological processes as we interact with our environment. Therefore, they support the view that mind and brain are not separate but integrated. On the one hand, how we behave impacts the biology of our brains. On the other hand, there are biological processes that are necessary for our thoughts, feelings, and behaviors. Neurotransmitters (chemicals that transmit impulses between nerves) and hormones (chemicals that stimulate or inhibit activity of target organs) are essential parts of these biological processes. These chemical substances play a role in the pain experience. The neurotransmitter serotonin directly transmits and modulates pain sensations. It also plays a role in anxiety and mood. The neurotransmitter norepinephrine is involved in anxiety, arousal, memory, and mood. It is also the principal neurotransmitter of the sympathetic nervous system.

The sympathetic nervous system transmits nerve impulses including those involved in pain. The fact that these neurotransmitters are part of both the mechanism for pain and the mechanism for emotions might mean that there is a direct biological link between a person's pain and his or her anxiety and depression. Unlike Ann, who became depressed in "reaction" to her pain and the loss of her hand, others might develop depression because their pain directly changes the chemicals needed to maintain a happy mood. In addition, the brain produces its own painkillers (analgesics) called endorphins. Furthermore, hormones that are produced in our brains activate our stress response systems, including the release of cortisol from the adrenal glands in our abdomens. Stress and pain mutually interact. Pain is a stressor; stress exacerbates pain.

Although our increasing understanding of the chemistry of the nervous system will result in better pain control, nonaddictive medications are presently available that are effective for chronic pain, but we do not know how they work. We use antidepressants (really a misnomer because they treat more than depression) that affect serotonin and norepinephrine to treat pain. Gabapentin, a seizure medication, is useful for neuropathic pain, that is, pain resulting from nerve injury, as opposed to nociceptic, or tissue damage, pain.

Obviously, we need to learn more about the chemistry of our brains. In particular, understanding the placebo effect is key to unlocking the puzzle of pain. The placebo (Latin root *placére*—I will please) is inactive but still causes an effect. This is amazing. Here is another example of the power of the mind and its integration with the brain. Just taking into our bodies a substance that we believe will relieve our pain can cause pain relief. Therefore, it is the power of expectation. There was some data that explained the placebo effect being due to the activation of the brain's endorphins. Other studies have not supported this. Therefore, we still do not know the biology of the placebo effect. Because of its safety and ability to relieve pain, it might be beneficial to use a placebo to treat pain. Although placebos are important for experimental studies, I advise against using a placebo to treat a person's post-traumatic pain. First, using a placebo requires that the physician deceive the patient. Second, it does not distinguish between psychogenic pain and pain related to tissue injury.

Phantom sensation is another fascinating phenomenon that supports the essential role of the brain in the pain experience. Many people who have undergone amputations still sense the presence of the missing body part.

In addition, if a limb has been amputated, movement of the missing limb can still be experienced. Phantom sensation is not a disease. Only education about this phenomenon is necessary. However, a smaller percentage of amputees actually experience pain in reference to the missing part of their body. This is a devastating disorder. How can this be? We usually talk about pain in regard to a place in our bodies. My leg hurts. I feel this terrible pain in my arm. However, it appears that one does not need a particular body part to experience pain. Does phantom limb pain indicate that we need only a brain to generate pain? Dr. Melzack thinks so. Although it does not replace his gate control theory, he recently proposed a *neuromatrix theory.* This theory explains how pain originates in the brain. This is the opposite of the specificity theory that attributed bodily injury as the entire cause for pain.

By placing this emphasis on learned behavior, thought, emotion, the placebo effect, and phantom pain, it appears that I am saying that pain is "all in your head." We usually understand this phrase to mean that the pain is only imagined, that is, a fantasy. Nevertheless, pain can be real and still be "in your head." In the introduction to this book, Dr. Simon remarks, "Without the brain to interpret certain signals from our bodies (and from the brain itself), there would be no pain." In this chapter, I demonstrate how the mind and brain are essential to the pain experience. This does not invalidate your suffering as a post-traumatic pain patient but rather helps you to understand what causes and maintains your suffering. Through knowledge we gain control.

Pain is real. The most valid dolorimetry, or method of measuring the intensity of pain, is to ask the person how much pain he or she is experiencing. Although we have the technology of X-rays, CAT scans, MRIs, and PET scans, the person experiencing the pain is the only "instrument" that is truly able to measure its intensity, frequency, and characteristics. Nevertheless, we physicians may sometimes doubt the pain reports of our patients. When a doctor tells his or her patient, "I have all the test results and there is nothing wrong," the patient thinks, "My doctor doesn't believe me. My pain means there is something wrong. If there is 'nothing wrong,' my doctor is saying I should not have any pain." This statement invalidates the patient's pain experience.

Doubting a patient's pain generates no treatment; underestimating the severity of pain produces inadequate treatment. Being true to the Hippocratic principle of "First, do no harm," physicians are concerned that their patients might become addicted to narcotic analgesic medication. Therefore, some physicians might underestimate the severity of the patient's pain. Underestimation of pain, and concern about potential addiction, results in underdosing of medication, especially in regard to acute traumatic pain.

The statement "None of the tests found any reason for your pain" is not much better. This statement validates the patient's pain but gives him or her something to worry about. This only increases the patient's anxiety. The patient worries and wonders, "Isn't pain a danger signal for an illness that might harm or kill me? Since I'm having pain, and my doctor cannot find the cause, aren't I still in danger?" In order to address this concern, we must distinguish between acute pain and chronic pain. Acute pain does "sound an alarm"; chronic pain, such as persistent post-traumatic pain, is the "alarm" going haywire. In acute pain, a diagnosis of the cause leads to a quick treatment that usually removes the danger. For example, the surgeon excises an inflamed appendix that might have burst without the surgery. In regard to post-traumatic pain, the physician sutures the wound to stop the bleeding and promote healing. In addition, he or she prescribes antibiotics to prevent infection and opioid analgesics to turn off the pain "alarm." In acute pain, opioid analgesics are beneficial because they relieve the pain that would otherwise inhibit the patient's mobility, and thus interfere with healing and promote the development of disability. In chronic pain, the "alarm" continues to ring, constantly or intermittently, although there is no danger or threat.

The best approach is one in which the physician neither dismisses, doubts, nor underestimates a patient's pain and says, "I am sorry that you are suffering with pain. Let's work together so that you can control, master, and obtain relief from this pain." This intervention is validating, reassuring, and collaborating. It also emphasizes "control," a factor that is essential to mastering pain.

Nothing in life has a 100-percent certainty except, as the saying goes, "death and taxes." Likewise, no medical test is 100-percent accurate. False-positive results occur when the test indicates that something exists that actually does not. It is a false positive when someone is diagnosed with having a disorder—for example, post-traumatic pain—when he or she is unaffected. Therefore, a person might report experiencing pain when he or she actually does not. Yes, even the most valid dolorimeter—the patient—may give a false-positive result.

Although it is rare, people may fake pain. There are two forms of faking or falsely reporting pain—malingering and factitious disorder (Münchausen's syndrome). Since these conditions are the exception, the best approach is to accept the pain as real. Nevertheless, there are certain situations where malingering and factitious disorder need to be considered.

Malingering is sometimes confused with psychogenic pain. (See "Diagnosis" on page 92.) In both malingering and psychogenic pain, there are no objective findings to support the degree of pain that is reported. For example, there is no tissue damage. Unlike the psychogenic pain patient who experiences real pain, the malingerer falsely reports pain that does not exist. The malingerer also might exaggerate the impairment of his or her functioning due to an actual injury, inflict an injury upon himself or herself, or fake an injury. The malingerer's sole purpose is to obtain *secondary gain,* for example, a financial benefit, or to shirk his or her responsibilities. Secondary gain—being cared for, being dependent—may also be a reinforcement (operant conditioning) for post-traumatic pain. Psychogenic pain is similar to *conversion disorder.* Conversion disorder is a dysfunction of voluntary movement (for example, paralysis of one's arm) or the senses (for example, temporary blindness) that can be viewed either as having no neurological explanation or as being produced as a compromise for an internal psychological conflict. Conversion was a common aspect of "shell shock" (the name used for the disorder we now call PTSD) in World War I among the American, British, French, and German combatants. A classic conversion disorder in a soldier was paralysis of his legs that developed in the heat and horror of battle. This symptom solved his unconscious psychological conflict, that is, his need to be brave and fight versus his fear of being killed. Furthermore, it was his fear that caused him not to rescue his buddy from being killed by the enemy. His paralysis allowed him to consciously believe that he really was brave but that he was unable to save his buddy because he could not walk. The benefit that one derives from no longer having the distress of the unconscious psychological conflict is called *primary gain.* Real pain without any injury also can provide primary gain. Thus, some pain sufferers might have the root of their pain deep in their unconscious.

We do not usually see pure psychogenic pain disorders or conversion disorders in modern day United States. In this day and age, conversion pain and psychogenic pain are more likely seen among people of devel-

DIAGNOSIS

Pain Disorder

Features	Associated with psychological factors.	Associated with with both psychological factors and general medical condition.	Associated with general medical condition.
Alternate Name	Psychogenic pain disorder.	None.	None.
Type of Symptom	Pain in any part of the body.		
Psychological Reason for Symptoms	To resolve internal psychological conflict.	Both psychological and general medical conditions have a role in the onset, severity, exacerbation, or maintenance of the pain.	None.
Aware of Reason	No, an unconscious process.	May or may not have insight about psychological factors.	Not applicable.
Reality of Pain	Real.	Real.	Real.
Production of Symptom	Not intentional.	Produced by injury or general medical condition.	
Altered Body Tissue	No.	Yes.	Yes.

DIAGNOSIS		
Psychological Disorder		
Conversion Disorder	Malingering	Factitious Disorder
None.	None.	Münchausen's syndrome.
Voluntary motor system (for example paralysis) or sensory (for example, blindness, loss of sensation).	Any symptom.	Any symptom.
To resolve internal psychological conflict.	An external incentive (for example, financial gain or avoidance of responsibility).	Need to be in the sick role.
No, an unconscious process.	Yes.	No.
Real.	Feigned (unless an exaggeration of an actual symptom or symptom is self-inflicted).	Feigned (unless symptom is self-inflicted).
Not intentional.	Intentional.	Intentional.
No.	No, unless self-inflicted.	No, unless self-inflicted.

oping countries. For example, a woman from an African country, who was grieving the death of her six-month-old child, dreamed that her face was being battered by people who angrily blamed her for her child's death. When she awoke she felt intense pain throughout her face that she hadn't experienced prior to her dream.

Some people with actual tissue injury might experience persistence of their pain because of an unconscious meaning for it, which might have originated in childhood. In his classic article, "'Psychogenic Pain' and the Pain Prone Patient," George Engel, a noted psychiatrist and internist, observed that certain people as adults were prone to use pain for psychological regulation because, as children, "aggression, suffering, and pain played an important role in early family relationships," including their being physically or verbally abused. These adults learned early in their lives that pain was a punishment for guilt. A study with a large number of patients supported this association between abuse in childhood and psychogenic pain later in life. Another study demonstrated that 64 percent of women with chronic pelvic pain had been sexually abused as children. This percentage of childhood sexual abuse was significantly greater than the percentage in the comparison group of patients who did not have pelvic pain. People who have undergone psychological trauma in childhood are more likely to be vulnerable to trauma as an adult. Thus, a comprehensive pain evaluation by a doctor should include asking about past traumatic experiences. For some people with post-traumatic pain, the road to recovery will include exploring and overcoming the known trauma of the past.

POST-TRAUMATIC STRESS DISORDER

"Oh, no! I'm going to die!" At twenty-six years old, Bob had everything to look forward to in his life. He was engaged to be married. His fiancée and he were making plans for the future—where they would live, how many children they would have, how they would each advance in their careers. Wham! All of sudden! Unexpectedly, a tractor trailer ran a red light, smashed into his car, and propelled the crumbled wreck off the road. He remembered yelling out, "Oh, no! I'm going to die!" as he caught a glimpse of the truck barreling down on him just before the impact.

Bob was alive, but as the fire rescue unit extricated him from his compressed car he felt very frightened and helpless. Although he was treated at a local hospital for a fractured left arm and multiple cuts from the shattered glass, no one attended to his emotional wounds. In the aftermath of the accident, he not only suffered arm, neck, and back pain but also had recurrent nightmares and distressing intrusive thoughts about the accident. Whenever he heard an emergency vehicle siren he startled, became anxious, and felt his heart race. He avoided talking about the accident and felt numb. When he was forced to relate what had happened, he had difficulty recalling the details. Most of the time he felt detached and without feelings for his fiancée. Some of the time he became irritable and screamed at her in anger. Initially, he refused to get into a car. When he finally did travel in a car as a passenger, he nervously glanced in all directions and became fearful if a truck was even in his vicinity. He seesawed between being emotionally numb without experiencing any pain and being intensely anxious with excruciating pain. The endless nights of difficulty falling asleep resulted in progressively worsening fatigue that added to his inability to concentrate. His lack of desire and his pain curtailed his activities. His life was shattered, and he no longer had any sense of the future.

Bob suffered from post-traumatic stress disorder (PTSD) and post-traumatic pain. Although PTSD and post-traumatic pain are separate disorders, it is not surprising to find them occurring together after trauma. Like post-traumatic pain, PTSD may develop after a person is physically injured. In a study, 80 percent of Vietnam combat veterans with PTSD reported experiencing chronic pain. Although a veterans' pain clinic only measured a PTSD rate of 10 percent among its patients, other research studies have shown that 50 to 100 percent of pain center patients may also suffer from PTSD. A study measured a 15-percent rate of PTSD among patients suffering facial pain of unknown origin. On the one hand, 21 percent of PTSD patients also suffered from fibromyalgia (see Chapter 3) according to a study. On the other hand, 56 percent of patients suffering with fibromyalgia also had PTSD-like symptoms in another study. This latter study also demonstrated that the fibromyalgia patients with PTSD-like symptoms had significantly greater levels of pain, emotional distress, interference with life, and disability. In another study, 34.7 percent of injured workers reported symptoms consistent with the diagnosis of PTSD. Based on a number of studies, the average rate of PTSD among motor-vehicle accident survivors who had received medical attention for their physical injuries is 29.5 percent.

What is PTSD? When you ask this question, you often receive many inaccurate answers. "Isn't it a rather recent disorder that is seen in Vietnam veterans?" "It's a legal diagnosis." "It's the symptoms that people make up to be in the victim role." "A war illness." "People use it to sue." The truth is that as long ago as ancient times, there have been literary descriptions of what we now call PTSD. Although some people doubt its validity, PTSD is a real disorder that has been described in the scientific literature in the United States since 1871. Furthermore, there is an abundance of scientific data and research documenting the clinical picture, epidemiology, psychobiology, and treatment of PTSD. Although the term PTSD was coined in 1980 for the third edition of the *American Psychiatric Association Diagnostic and Statistical Manual of Mental Disorders* (DSM-III), the forerunner of PTSD, "gross stress reaction," appeared in the first DSM in 1952. Although many associate PTSD only with war, a civilian type of PTSD was officially recognized in the initial DSM.

During each of the wars fought by the United States beginning with World War I, physicians acknowledged that the horrors of war caused terrible psychological wounds. Despite learning this lesson during the course of each war, the medical field forgot what it had learned each time peace was declared. Therefore, it was necessary to relearn about psychological trauma during the next war. Finally, the political activism that flourished during and after the Vietnam War era was a force that propelled our nation to accept combat PTSD once and for all. A prolonged and difficult struggle resulted in the United States Congress passing legislature that funded programs to treat veterans suffering with PTSD.

PTSD is a mental disorder that develops after exposure to an event that is life threatening or threatens physical injury or results in actual physical injury. The characteristic symptoms of PTSD that develop after a traumatic event are grouped into three clusters: 1) reexperiencing of the trauma, 2) avoidance of cues of the trauma and numbness of feelings 3) hyperarousal. (See the "PTSD Symptom Checklist" on page 98.)

Despite the progress toward the recognition of combat PTSD, I see many nonveteran patients with PTSD who are revictimized by nonbelievers who doubt the validity of this disorder, dispute the link between this disorder and a traumatic event, and discount the suffering of these patients. This battle against accepting PTSD as a biological disorder dates back to the 1800s in Britain when railroad travel was popular and compensation laws were enacted. Over a span of about thirty years, physicians debated whether individuals claiming to be injured in railway accidents were malingering ("compensation neurosis"), impaired because of direct physical injury ("railway spine"), or suffering from a psychological disorder caused by experiencing the traumatic accident ("nervous shock"). Despite all our scientific knowledge, this battle still rages. The mindset of many insurers, attorneys, and judges is biased toward believing that a person is being fraudulent whenever he or she claims to have PTSD. Even some relatives and friends of the PTSD sufferer expect him or her to just "snap out of it" because they believe it is not a real disorder.

I predict that our national tragedy on September 11, 2001, will change this negative attitude in our society about PTSD. Almost all of us have experienced some degree of "symptoms" such as anxiety, fear, insomnia, nightmares, and distressing intrusive thoughts, in response to the 9–11 terrorist attacks even if we only witnessed these events through television. Therefore, having this experience may engender empathy for those who suffer from PTSD. If a person is unable to sleep or has nightmares just as a result of watching this disaster on television, he or she is better able to imagine what it must have been like for those who were at ground zero and survived. If just reading about the gruesomeness of the rescue and recovery efforts stirs a feeling of horror, we are better able to imagine what it has been like for the rescue and recovery workers.

Nevertheless, traumatic stress—a natural, human reaction of short duration in response to a catastrophic event—is what most people experienced in response to the 9–11 traumatic events. In the United States, about 61 percent of men and about 51 percent of women will be exposed to at least one traumatic event during their lifetimes. Unfortunately, motor vehicle accidents, industrial accidents, violent assaults, and other traumatic events happen. The good news is that most of those who are exposed to traumatic events do not develop PTSD. Although many might experience traumatic stress, only an average of about 8 percent of men and about 20 percent of women who experience a traumatic event develop PTSD. The percentage of people who develop PTSD depends on the type of traumatic event. For example, 34 percent of the survivors who were in or around the Murrah Federal Building in Oklahoma City

PTSD SYMPTOM CHECKLIST

If any of the following symptoms have occurred and persisted after the traumatic event that is related to your pain, inform your physician.

- I am on the alert that something threatening might happen.
- I am unable to remember some of the important parts of the event.
- I easily jump or startle.
- I experience distressing recurrent and intrusive recollections of the event.
- I feel detached or estranged from others.
- I experience intense emotional distress when I am reminded of the event.
- I feel irritable and/or have angry outbursts.
- I find myself acting or feeling as if the event is happening again.
- I have difficulty concentrating.
- I have difficulty falling asleep and/or staying asleep.
- I have physical reactions like a rapid heartbeat, sweating, and/or trembling when I am reminded of the event.
- I have recurrent distressing dreams about the event.
- I make an effort to avoid or I do avoid activities, places, and/or people that arouse recollections of the event.
- I make an effort to avoid or I do avoid thinking, feeling, and/or talking about the event.
- I think that somehow my future will be cut short.
- My interest or participation in activities that I have liked has greatly diminished.
- My loving feelings for others are restricted.

at the time of the bomb explosion have developed PTSD. The bad news is that once PTSD develops and goes untreated, it can chronically persist for 40 percent of those who have the disorder. People suffering with PTSD are six times more likely to attempt suicide than people without PTSD. Therefore, early detection and treatment of PTSD is very important to prevent chronicity, disability, and suicide.

What is our present explanation for the development of PTSD? Upon exposure to a life-threatening event, we, like other animals, respond with a "fight-flight-freeze" reaction. We either mobilize to counter the threat, flee to safety, or freeze in a state of fear. Our sympathetic nervous systems play a central role in this reaction. This is a very adaptive survival mechanism. However, if you are a person who develops PTSD, this experience causes a conditioned fear through the process of classical conditioning. Some factors, such as previous trauma or having disorders of anxiety or depression in your family, may have placed you at risk for developing this disordered response. Your hormonal stress response system activates but might turn off prematurely and, thus, not limit other biological mechanisms. Although conditioned fear is a rapid, unconscious process involving the amygdala (an almond-shaped structure in the limbic system, that is, the primitive part of our brains), conscious thought appears to also play a role in your developing PTSD. During the "fight-flight-freeze" reaction, the outpouring of adrenaline (epinephrine) in your brain causes a stronger memory consolidation of the images of the traumatic event. Your cognitive appraisal can result in viewing the event either as a challenge or as an extreme threat without any escape. The latter meaning provokes you to feel intense fear, helplessness, and/or horror.

Once you are no longer in danger, the conditioned fear causes you to automatically behave as if the danger were still present. Just like Pavlov's dogs who salivated upon hearing the bell, you react to cues and reminders of the traumatic event that no longer exists. In addition, you develop an attentional bias—a sensitivity toward traumalike stimuli—that results in physiological and psychological reactivity when you are exposed to such stimuli. Furthermore, your mind is unable to process the memories of the traumatic event. Thus, you experience a barrage of distressing, repetitious, intrusive thoughts. Sometimes you might even feel as if you are reliving the traumatic experience as you have a flashback of intense sounds, smells, visions, and/or bodily reactions. Even dreaming, which is a way for us to process our thoughts and conflicts, provides no relief to you. Instead, you experience nightmares. This repeated replay of the trauma without any resolution might bc responsible for causing an emotionally charged, indelible "imprint" in your brain that leads you to develop chronic PTSD.

Avoidance opposes experiencing these intense thoughts, emotions, and physiologic reactivity. You consciously and intentionally avoid what you fear, for example, by deliberately not getting into a car even weeks after being injured in a motor vehicle accident. When you avoid people, places, and things that remind you of the trauma, you feel better or, at least, do not feel worse. Thus, your avoidance behavior becomes reinforced through the process of operant conditioning (avoidance learning). In addition, your mind unconsciously and automatically avoids through the process of dissociation. Memories, thoughts, and emotions are separated from one another. This results in your becoming emotionally numb, detached, and estranged. You are present with your loved ones but do not feel emotionally engaged. You have difficulty recalling aspects of your trauma that moments before appeared so vivid in your mind. Your memories about what actually happened become fragmented. Your PTSD becomes a seesawing between reexperiencing the trauma and being numb. There is insufficient serotonin in your brain synapses to dampen the symptoms that you are experiencing. The possibility of your feeling survivor guilt and blaming yourself (known as attribution) only adds to your woes.

The psychobiological processes of PTSD are tempered by social support at the time of the trauma and during recovery. Thus, the nature of the immediate professional interventions and the support of your family and friends might be variables in the development and maintenance of your PTSD. The following is another example of how the environment influences our brains.

"I always feel headaches and fear." Ever since the tornado during which flying debris struck twenty-five-year-old Sally on the head and caused her to have a temporary loss of consciousness, she has been experiencing frequent headaches and fear that another tornado will happen. She is very hypervigilant and constantly listens to the twenty-four-hour weather station. In addition, she has manifested avoidance behavior, diminished interest, estrangement from others, exaggerated startle reaction, inability to tolerate noise or bright lights, intrusive distressing recollections of the tornado, irritability, lapses of memory, nightmares, numbed feelings, and poor concentration. Whenever there are wind gusts, she becomes very anxious and starts to sweat.

When a person's trauma involves a direct blow to the skull or violent movement of the head, the psychiatrist considers whether the person suffers from either PTSD or traumatic brain injury (see Chapter 4: Hidden Concussions) or both of these disorders. Traumatic brain injury may range from post-concussion syndrome and subtle cognitive impairments to severe dementia.

Trauma, fear, and pain have a lot in common. Classical conditioning, operant conditioning, learned helplessness, cognitive appraisal, attribution, catastrophizing, attentional bias, and the same neurochemicals are involved in PTSD and in pain. Another link between PTSD and pain may involve *endorphin,* the brain's opiatelike painkiller. A study measured an increased secretion of endorphin in patients with PTSD who were exposed to reminders of their traumas. Based on this data and the phenomenon of inescapable shock (learned helplessness), Bessel van der Kolk, Roger Pitman, and their colleagues have postulated a biological explanation for the seesawing between the reexperiencing and numbing that occurs in PTSD. According to this theory, PTSD is like an addiction in which numbing is due to an increase of the brain's endorphin level along with a transient depletion of certain neurotransmitters, and reexperiencing is "withdrawal," that is, a lowering of the endorphin level in the brain and a hypersensitivity of norepinephrine neurons.

PTSD and post-traumatic pain are reciprocally reinforcing. PTSD worsens bodily pain; bodily pain worsens PTSD. Your pain triggers traumatic memories and physiologic reactivity. The physiologic reactivity heightens your pain sensitivity. You fear being re-traumatized and reinjured. You overestimate the probability of the traumatic event reoccurring and your being reinjured. You fear falling asleep lest you have nightmares. When you do finally doze off, your pain awakens you. Lack of sufficient sleep saps your energy and takes a toll on your overall health. And so it goes—back and forth, around and around. You discover you are in a state of helplessness. Therefore, it is absolutely necessary to be treated for PTSD when it is present along with post-traumatic pain in order to break this cycle of reciprocal reinforcement.

HOPE FOR the post-traumatic pain sufferer includes focusing on the psychiatric aspects of pain, especially the role of post-traumatic stress disorder (PTSD). The International Association for the Study of Pain (IASP) recognized the importance of the psychiatric aspects of pain when it defined pain as an unpleasant sensory and emotional experience associated with actual or potential tissue damage or described in terms of such damage. The psychiatrist is the physician with the specialized medical training and expertise to diagnose and ultimately treat the mental disorders, including PTSD, anxiety disorders, major depressive disorder, dementia, and alcohol and drug abuse or dependence that may be associated with post-traumatic pain. Therefore, a psychiatric evaluation is a necessary part of a comprehensive assessment of a person suffering with chronic post-traumatic pain. In addition, it is advisable that some patients with acute post-traumatic pain be seen for a psychiatric consultation in order to assess the need for early psychiatric intervention that would prevent complications, chronic pain, and disability. Psychotherapy is often a necessary and beneficial part of the management of post-traumatic pain. Finally, it is best to diagnosis and treat the mental illness associated with pain, especially PTSD, as early as possible.

SUGGESTED READINGS

Allen, J.G. *Coping with Trauma: A Guide to Self-Understanding.* Washington, DC: American Psychiatric Press, Inc., 1995.

Greist, John H., et al. *Posttraumatic Stress Disorder: A Guide.* Madison, WI: Madison Institute of Medicine, 2000.

To order this guide, call Madison Institute of Medicine at 608-827-2470 or visit their Web site at www.miminc.org.

HELPFUL WEB SITES AND ORGANIZATIONS

American Pain Foundation
http://www.painfoundation.org

American Psychiatric Association
http://www.psych.org

Anxiety Disorders Association of America
http://www.adaa.org

This is a professional and consumer organization. You can get a pamphlet on PTSD. Visit their Web site or call 301-231-9350.

Englewood Hospital and Medical Center

http://www.englewoodhospital.com

This is a very user-friendly Web site for health-care consumers that provides a variety of services. Click on "Health Information/Library" and then on "Health Consumer/Patient Web Sites" or "Medical Web Sites" for links to many excellent health-related Web sites.

International Society for Traumatic Stress Studies

http://www.istss.org

This is a professional society of traumatic stress experts that has resources for the public.

MedicineNet

http://www.medicinenet.com

A consumer-oriented Web site that offers features on diseases and treatments, a pharmacy section, medical tests and procedures, etc.

Medline Plus

http://www.nlm.nih.gov/medlineplus

Health information from the National Library of Medicine. Those who are interested in participating in research may access information about clinical trials by clicking on "ClinicalTrials.gov" on the Medline Plus homepage.

Meland Foundation

http://www.melandfoundation.org

A non-profit organization created to provide access to health-care information.

PTSD Alliance

http://www.ptsdalliance.org

This is a group of professional and advocacy organizations that have joined forces to provide educational resources to individuals diagnosed with PTSD and their loved ones; those at risk for developing PTSD; and medical, health-care, and other frontline professionals.

PART

2

WHAT CAN I DO ABOUT IT?

THIS PART is all about choice. You can choose to stay as you are—suffering with disabling post-traumatic pain—or you can choose to take charge of your condition and try to improve it by using one or more of the therapeutic treatments described in the following chapters.

TRADITIONAL AND ALTERNATIVE MEDICINE

In choosing methods of treatment, you have available not only traditional, conventional medical treatments but also alternative, complementary treatments.

Traditional medicine—surgery, physical rehabilitation, psychotherapy, and drug therapy—is based upon scientific principles that began in ancient Greece with Hippocrates. Traditional medical treatments have undergone rigorous experimental testing and study. Those treatments that are repeatedly found to be effective and safe are maintained and utilized by physicians, and those that fail to produce better-than-average results are discontinued.

Alternative treatments have no such scientific tradition. However, some of these therapies are based upon an ancient history of effective use. Herbal therapy, for example, was known to prehistoric man, and acupuncture and Ayurvedic medicine have been practiced in the East since ancient times.

Just recently, medical practitioners in the United States have begun to examine alternative treatment methods through scientific inquiry, and the White House Commission on Alternative and Complementary Medicine has been established under the direction of Dr. James Gordon, a Harvard University psychiatrist.

The three principal authors of this book are all traditional medical practitioners. Nevertheless, we encourage our patients to use all methods of treatment that may help them, including alternative treatments, as long as we consider these treatments safe. The contributors we have selected to describe these alternative methods of treatment in the chapters that follow have years of experience with their individual programs, and their suggestions and explanations can be trusted to provide you with commonsense approaches to relief from post-traumatic pain.

CHOICES OF TREATMENT

Chapter 7: Knowledge Is Power, by Dr. Simon, encourages you to inform yourself about both traditional and alternative treatment programs and to feel the power that this knowledge provides in the battle against post-traumatic pain syndrome.

Chapter 8: Prescriptions to Treat Chronic Pain, by Dr. Ehrlich, summarizes some of his wide-ranging knowledge of pain medications and their side effects.

In Chapter 9: Treating Your Symptoms after a Concussion, Dr. Sadwin describes ways of treating forty physical and emotional symptoms of concussion.

Alternative therapy is the subject of Chapter 10: Proof of Alternative Therapies, by radiologist Andrew Newberg, M.D. Dr. Newberg discusses the fact that although alternative therapies may have no scientific basis, they do have a scientifically demonstrable effect on your brain in controlling pain: In other words, if you believe in your treatment, your belief itself becomes the treatment.

An innovative treatment for pain related to acupuncture and trigger-point therapy is discussed in Chapter 11: Acupuncture and Trigger-Point Therapy, by Jennifer Chu, M.D.

T'ai chi master Jano Cohen is the author of Chapter 12: Bodywork, which describes hands-on treatments such as Rolfing, Reiki, movement therapy, and other techniques designed to relieve pain and improve physical function.

In Chapter 13: Eat Better to Feel Better, psychologist and weight-loss expert Gloria Horwitz explains how you can use nutrition to combat post-traumatic pain syndrome. She describes how the stress of recovering from trauma can disturb patterns in eating behavior, how these patterns create additional stress, and how to replace them with healthy habits.

Rheumatologist Sharon Kolasinski, M.D., discusses herbal treatments of pain in Chapter 14: Herbal Therapy for Chronic Pain.

In Chapter 15: Ayurvedic Medicine, Arvind Chopra, M.D., describes the ancient treatment of pain by Ayurvedic medicine.

The ways in which chiropractic treatment is used to treat spinal conditions that cause pain are described in Chapter 16: Chiropractic Care, by Bruce Pfleger, Ph.D. In this chapter, Dr. Pfleger explains the theory of chiropractic care and how it differs from traditional medical therapy.

Yoga is the subject of Chapter 17. Author Marion Garfinkel, Ed.D., is a master of this ancient art, which can decrease both stress and pain.

In the final chapter, Chapter 18: Disability versus Impairment, orthopedic surgeon Barry Snyder, M.D., discusses how you can return to work and a productive life despite physical impairment.

But first, as a summary of one patient's successful experience in using several of these alternative therapies, the following is "A Doctor's Own Story of Healing" by Elizabeth Michel, M.D. In this account, Dr. Michel tells how, after traditional medical treatment, she chose alternative therapies to help relieve her pain and stress, and how, with the aid of these therapies—plus a lot of hope and perseverance—she successfully rehabilitated her body and regained the joy of living.

William H. Simon, M.D.

A DOCTOR'S OWN STORY OF HEALING

ELIZABETH MICHEL, M.D.

Although doctors are said to make the worst patients—we tend to be reluctant to admit that we could use some help ourselves—my professional training has enabled me to study what trauma specialists have been learning and to apply some of this information to my own recovery.

My career choice was an important aspect of my personality structure, which helped me to survive many challenges, including violence in my childhood home. But my personality was ill equipped to deal with the consequences of a serious accident. Stubborn dedication to working hard on my recovery could take me closer to what I could reasonably accomplish, but it got in the way of letting go of what I could not. As you will see, letting go is by no means the same as giving up.

Your own personality has no doubt helped you to endure some challenges unique to your own life. At the same time, it might be preventing you from living your post-accident life as fully and contentedly as you could.

Learning to Walk

When I came home from the hospital, my baby would not even look at me. But the next morning, my husband, Arnie, brought him to me with a bottle of milk, and he began to warm up to me once again. In the evenings, Arnie and my sister would lift me out of my wheelchair and set me on the kitchen floor so that I could play with the baby as he crawled around. Arnie joked about who would walk first. But I still felt deep anguish over not being able to mother my baby properly.

A few weeks later, I was given new, somewhat lighter casts. Each morning after Arnie and the children left, I slid down several steps to the living room on my backside and pulled myself up again at the piano. Years later, I read a quote from Victor Hugo: "Music expresses that which cannot be put into words and cannot remain silent." I was in agony, but I could not speak of it. No one wanted to know, least of all myself.

Four months after my accident, as soon as I could walk well enough, I went back to my part-time job. I was not conscious of it until later, but I was asserting, "If I can take care of patients, there's nothing wrong with me." Denial serves well when survival is at stake, but in the long run it becomes destructive. Fortunately, the work was easy; most of my patients were healthy college students with minor infections.

During this time, I was still having pain when I walked, and it became clear that my right tibia, the large bone between the knee and the ankle, had not healed properly. My orthopedist told me that he could break the bone surgically and reset it, or I could live with it the way it was.

I was terrified that I would be crippled if I left the tibia uncorrected, but I also was terrified of having more surgery and more pain. Arnie was against the operation; he said that it would inconvenience him again. Later, we understood that he too was reacting to trauma—he had nearly been left alone with two tiny children, and now he had a mate who was more impaired than either of us was willing to admit. But at the time, his selfishness hurt and angered me. I began to have sexual fantasies about a young man I knew who was very strong and athletic—exactly what I no longer was but yearned to be. I started to feel that I was going crazy. After consulting a second orthopedist, I decided to schedule the surgery, but I became depressed and began to see a psychotherapist.

Letting Go

A few weeks after the operation on my right leg, I returned to a part-time position. But I saw clearly that I was less well than the students I was caring for. I was in pain, depressed, and, it turned out, quite anemic.

Once my anemia was treated with iron supplements, I lost a strange craving I had developed the year before: I had been chewing ice. I had even cracked three molars and needed complicated repairs. I was deeply ashamed of my secret "addiction" and didn't tell my dentist. But the medically obvious—that I had *pica,* a common symptom of iron deficiency—never occurred to me. My dental self-destruction illustrates how easily stress can provoke problems not directly caused by the accident.

I realized that I was not ready to work even part-time, and I resigned. Although I felt devalued and frightened by the loss of my ability to support myself, the slower pace of my life was a relief. The rhythm of my new life gave me a chance to listen to parts of myself that had closed down, either long ago in my childhood or recently in the aftermath of my accident.

My therapist specialized in Jungian psychotherapy, in which dreams and the expressive arts are used to restore emotional and spiritual balance. She encouraged me to write poetry and to draw images from my dreams, and I enrolled in a poetry class at my local community college.

I also bought a book on weight training and a set of weights and started using them at home. And I kept on walking. The pain in my legs did not go away, but it slowly improved.

Bioenergetics Therapy

Several years after my accident, I saw an announcement for a weekly women's bioenergetic group. Bioenergetic analysis is a body-oriented approach to psychotherapy. Its founder, Dr. Alexander Lowen, was a pioneer in exploring the connection between mind and body. He believed that emotions that cannot be expressed are held in the human body in recognizable patterns of muscle tension, and he devised exercises to release muscle tension by combining movement and the expression of feeling. Some of his ideas are now outdated, but his approach helped me to understand how psychological distress can cause physical problems.

In the women's bioenergetic group, I found a safe, nurturing environment for releasing some of the tension in my body. In 1988, eight years after my accident, I decided to enter the bioenergetic institute's professional four-year training program. One of the requirements of the training program was to undergo bioenergetic therapy.

In 1990, I was invited to give a seminar on accident trauma to my bioenergetic society. To prepare for my lecture, I searched through the existing medical and psychological literature on the psychological impact of accident trauma, but I turned up very little. However, one article that I did find on the subject began:

"There are at least three illnesses in the victim of physical trauma. The first two are the injury and its regular companion, a traumatic neurosis from the overwhelming experience of the accident and its emergency treatment. . . . The third illness consists of the emotional problems the patient was fighting at the time of his accident" (James L. Titchener, "Management and Study of Psychological Response to Trauma," *Journal of Trauma* 10 (11) (1970): 974–80).

I realized that I was still suffering from two forms of post-traumatic stress disorder (PTSD): one the result of the accident and the other a complex and lifelong result of childhood abuse. By understanding the symptoms of PTSD, I learned to take better care of myself with a combination of physical therapy and psychotherapy.

Relaxing and Overcoming Anxiety

At the start of my fourth year of bioenergetics training, I was asked to counsel patients for a few hours each week as part of a program at the hospital. I accepted—and immediately became ill with anxiety. Night after night, I couldn't sleep for more than a few hours. Soon I was exhausted, and my pain worsened.

In general, I do not like to take medications, but I knew that I needed more help. I consulted a psychiatrist and was given a prescription for an antidepressant. Almost immediately, my anxiety and depression began to lift, although I had some side effects, including a feeling of emotional numbness.

After a year and a half, it became clear that I would not be able to continue to care for patients without staying on an antidepressant. Although I enjoyed my work, I resigned because I did not want to continue to take medication.

Around this time, I enrolled in a pain-management program at my hospital. In eight weekly sessions and homework assignments, my classmates and I learned to recognize many of the automatic thoughts we had in response to daily events in our lives. We observed how these automatic thoughts often led to tension and anxiety, and we practiced forming alternative thoughts. For example, one morning my knees hurt more than usual, and my automatic thought was, "My pain is getting worse." My alternative thought was, "I'm just stiff because I've been sitting so long at the computer." My automatic thought, I noted, made me feel angry and fearful, while my alternative thought resulted in less anger and fear, as well as a determination to schedule my work more carefully.

I also began to undergo deep-tissue massage therapy. This was not covered by my health insurance, so it was expensive and made me feel uncomfortably self-indulgent. But it was remarkably helpful.

Yoga

Nine years ago, a new friend urged me to accompany her to a yoga class at the YMCA. Since that first class, I have been practicing yoga regularly.

Yoga has been uniquely helpful to me because it works every part of my body. It stretches as well as strengthens all my muscles. As yoga has relaxed my muscles, my breathing patterns have changed. Although at times I recognize that I am breathing with the shallow respirations that characterize fear, more often I enjoy the slower, fuller breaths of calm alertness.

In India it is said that yoga is only a preparation for meditation. After practicing yoga for a few years, I began to attend a weekly meditation group at my religious fellowship. There, I study Buddhist teachings, which keep me from feeling isolated, and the simple meditation techniques I practice there relax my body and deepen my breathing.

Adapting to Head Trauma

Fifteen years after my accident, I began to have painful headaches, so I went to see a neurologist. He began my appointment by saying, "Before we start to talk about your headaches, tell me how you've been in general." I answered, "Well, I've never had the same physical stamina since my accident, and I've never had the same emotional stamina, either."

As soon as I said this, my colleague launched into a lengthy educational talk on "mild" head trauma. He told me that in recent years it had become clear that nerve fibers in the brain are torn during mild head trauma of the sort I had had when I suffered a concussion during my accident. Some patients never again feel as strong emotionally, he said.

Evidence of mild organic damage can be hard to demonstrate in high-functioning individuals, and tests later given to me by a psychologist revealed nothing. But soon afterward, I read a book published for patients who have suffered mild head trauma, called *Coping with Mild Traumatic Brain Injury,* by Diane Roberts Stoler and Barbara Albers Hill. It contained helpful suggestions about how to organize daily activities in order to feel less distracted or overwhelmed by social stimulation.

Since I have learned about mild head trauma, I have continued to heal from post-traumatic stress disorder and chronic pain. Now I can enjoy more social stimulation and take on new challenges with less anxiety.

Living in the Present

Today, twenty-one years after my accident, I can feel some joy in how far I have come. Yes, I often have pain when I am on my legs, and I regularly have to sit down to rest. I can no longer do the mountain hiking I once enjoyed. Arnie loves India, but just thinking about climbing the steps to an ancient temple makes my legs ache, so now I love to stay at home when he goes away. For vacations together, we choose a quiet cabin where we can enjoy easy hiking and I can get plenty of sleep each night, unpressured by an itinerary.

Some things that I would like to do are still too stressful, and I choose my challenges carefully. Last year, when I was asked to join the board of an organization, I delayed my decision a couple of weeks to observe whether my anxiety increased, my sleep deteriorated, or my pain worsened as I thought about the new responsibilities. When I found that I could feel excited about this work without an increase in symptoms, I said yes.

My life will always be limited in some ways by my accident, but within those limits I go on learning to flourish. Now I try to live more in the present. Simple things, such as vegetables ripening in my garden, surprise me with happiness now. I have a much better sense of humor than I did before my accident. Although our marriage was tested by trauma, Arnie and I learned together that love can grow stronger through grief. My sons grew up resilient, and the baby who wouldn't look at me when I came home from the hospital calls often and says, "I love you, Mom," before he hangs up the phone in his dorm room 3,000 miles away.

What You Can Do

I am a fortunate accident survivor, and I offer the following recommendations with the understanding that others may have more difficulty in finding what they need than I did. Still, I hope that my story will encourage you to be creative as you look for ways to heal.

- Stay as physically active as you can. If you were not physically active before the accident, or if you feel that your pain is keeping you from returning to moderate forms of exercise such as walking, yoga, or swimming even after your doctor has given you permission to do so, consider working with a body-oriented psychotherapist to recover your body's innate desire to express its strength and flexibility.
- If you have symptoms of post-traumatic stress disorder, either from the accident itself or from your pre-accident life, be sure to work with a psychotherapist who is trained to treat trauma.
- If your injuries do not preclude it, try some yoga classes. Many community programs and gyms offer yoga classes at reasonable prices. Find a teacher with a gentle style and a flexible approach.
- Try to structure your life so that you have a quiet place and adequate hours for sleep. If your sleep is disturbed regularly by anxiety or nightmares, get professional help.
- You may need to change your expectations about what you should accomplish during your waking hours. Simplifying one's life generally brings more serenity.
- Attend a class or program in chronic pain management. Although you cannot hope to be cured of your pain in a class, you can learn how to cope with it.

- Practice an art or a craft that absorbs and soothes you. Do this for yourself, and try not to worry about the end result and whether other people will like it.
- After an accident, you may be sorely challenged to accept your own limitations and those of your physicians, your family, or even all of humanity. Learn from those who have emerged from their own suffering with new coping skills and increased compassion for others.
- Join a support group. Find a spiritual community where you feel comfortable. Do some volunteer work.
- Go places where you can learn that pain is inevitable in the course of human life.
- Go places where you can learn that love is more powerful than loss.

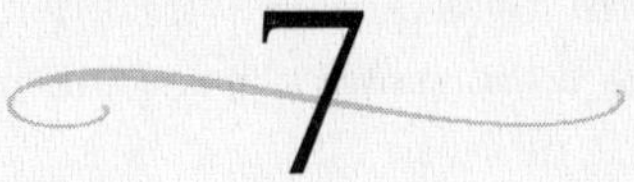

7

Knowledge Is Power

WILLIAM H. SIMON, M.D.

"Knowledge is power!" This statement made by Francis Bacon in 1597 is just as applicable today as it was 405 years ago. After having read Part One, you now know more about the causes of your post-traumatic pain. Do you feel any better? Do you need more help? That's what this section is all about—help and hope. You also have the power to choose how to help yourself get better.

We will assume that you don't need surgery—you've already had the surgery needed to treat your injuries, and you don't want any more operations, even if they were offered. Instead, you're ready to explore answers to the question "What can I do about it?" The chapters that follow will allow you to explore treatment options, both traditional and complementary (nontraditional or alternative medicine) for your post-traumatic pain syndrome.

We have gathered information from experts in many fields for your benefit. Please understand that we can't guarantee a "sure cure" for your particular problem. However, we do know that thousands of people with chronic pain have used one (or a combination of several) of these therapies with good results.

NEWS ABOUT ALTERNATIVE MEDICINE

In 1993, a report in the prestigious medical journal the *New England Journal of Medicine* stated that more than one-third of the patients they questioned used some form of alternative treatment. Americans in 1997 made 600 million office visits to providers of alternative medicine, spending $30 billion.

Harvard and Beth Israel Deaconess Medical Centers in Boston are using a $10 million grant to create the Harvard Medical School-Osher Institute for Research and Education in Complementary and Integrative Medical Therapies, the *Boston Globe* reported on May 1, 2001. The Office for Alternative Medicine has been established by The National Institutes of Health, in Bethesda, Maryland, to study some of the very techniques we are about to discuss in this part. Do these techniques work? Our patients tell us that they do, and as long as they are safe, we do not hesitate to recommend them to other patients.

THE PLACEBO EFFECT

Before we continue, we should explain that sometimes a patient feels better after treatment with a medicine or a procedure that has been proven to be inert (it has neither a positive nor a negative value). This phenomenon is called the "placebo effect." A placebo could be a sugar pill, for example, given to a certain set of patients who are told that they are receiving a strong pain medication. Another group of patients is actually given a strong pain medicine. An interview after the study is complete determines that a certain number of the patients who received the sugar pill experienced pain relief. This is known as the placebo effect.

There is nothing wrong with feeling better, and if any of the treatments that we will discuss (either traditional or complementary) make you feel well, so much the better. In other words, whether the treatment itself or the belief in the treatment improves your condition, the important thing to you is that you feel better. The National Institutes of Health, however, would want to know whether the treatment itself improved your condition or whether your belief in the effectiveness of the treatment is what helped you.

TRADITIONAL THERAPY

Before getting into the alternative treatments, let's spend some time talking about some traditional therapy. Since back pain is such a common finding in the post-traumatic pain syndrome, let us look at back pain.

Everybody gets a sore back now and then. (You take a shower, take an aspirin, and take a nap, and your back feels better. That's not a problem.) It becomes a problem when you have back pain every day—when you get up in the morning and you can barely get out of bed. At the end of the day, you feel as though someone is twisting a knife in your back. Every movement you make causes wracking pain in your back and/or in your leg(s). You can't sleep. Now, you have a problem!

The causes of back pain are numerous. The following are just a few: arthritis (degenerative, rheumatoid, and gouty), degenerative disc disease, herniated lumbar disc, spinal stenosis, spondylolysis, spondylolisthesis, spinal infection, spinal tumor, metastatic tumor, and nerve root scarring after an operation.

DIAGNOSTIC TESTS FOR BACK PAIN

You may be asked to take a number of diagnostic tests. X-rays are very helpful. They will show whether you have structural abnormalities in your spine, congenital (from birth) or degenerative (increasing with age). They will not show whether you have pain. More sophisticated studies may be required—CAT scan, MRI scan, myelogram, discogram, EMG, or blood studies. If you want to know more about this alphabet soup, read on.

The CAT Scan

CAT is short for computerized axial tomography. This diagnostic tool is a combination of an X-ray machine and a computer. X-rays show only bones or other calcified material. When you add a computer, you have "shades of gray," which show the noncalcified tissues—muscles, ligaments, nerves, and discs. A tomogram is a special type of X-ray that allows cross-sectional pictures of small sections of the body. The scan is performed by having you lie inside a large, round X-ray machine. There is no noise, no sensation at all. The pictures created are just like very detailed X-rays of very specific parts of your body, as specific as one single disc space. These pictures will demonstrate a lot of things, but they will not show pain. They will show anatomic or pathologic abnormalities, fractures, dislocations, degenerative joint disease, degenerative disc disease, herniated intervertebral discs, spinal stenosis, and/or tumors, but only an expert clinician can determine whether or not the findings are the cause of your back pain.

The Magnetic Resonance Imaging (MRI) Scan

An MRI (magnetic resonance imaging) scan is not an X-ray. As a matter of fact, it works using magnets and radiofrequency waves to produce a three-dimensional image of your spine. An MRI will show the good, the bad, and the ugly—but it still won't show the pain. The scanner can be a bit intimidating, but most modern scanners are "open" so that you won't become claustrophobic in a confined space. If you have the tendency for claustrophobia, always ask if the scanner is an "open" one before you report for the scan. Also, expect some banging noise. Don't be scared—they just can't shut the thing up. Sometimes you will be supplied with earphones with piped in music to cover the noise. All in all, it's not a bad experience.

The Myelogram

Now for the myelogram. This used to be the "gold standard" of spinal diagnostic studies of the spine. But it now takes a backseat to the MRI. In addition, it is an invasive study—someone has to stick a needle in your back. (I knew you wouldn't like that!) A radio opaque dye is injected into your spinal canal, then X-rays are taken as you are tilted up and down and as the dye moves up and down your spinal canal. The dye, which appears white on an X-ray plate, outlines the spinal nerves. If anything compresses these neural structures (disc herniation, fracture fragments, or tumor) a divot appears in the normally smooth appearance of the nerve roots or of the spinal cord. Often a CAT scan is performed with the dye in place to add a direct visualization to the indirect myelographic picture. The dye dissolves on its own, by the way. So no one has to stick you again to remove it. Usually there are no consequences following this study. Some people occasionally develop a headache from hell and have to stay flat in bed for twenty-four hours. If you have an allergy to iodine, don't take this test! The dye used in this procedure is an iodinated compound.

The Discogram

The discogram. Ah, the discogram. This is another invasive test. This time, the iodinated dye (make sure you tell the doctor if you have an allergy to iodine so that he can take precautions) is injected directly into the intervertebral disc. The diagnostic value of the test is measured in two ways. First, the pattern of the dye in the disc is evaluated, as captured on an X-ray. If there is disc degeneration or herniation, the dye will leak out of its central position through the cracks or tear in the disc. Second, the leaky disc will take more fluid volume than a normal disc, and the insertion of the dye in the appropriate disc will reproduce the pain you are complaining about. Now, you've located the pain source—maybe! Sometimes, two discs will cause the same pain; sometimes, the pain is not exactly like what you normally experience. But it happens to be the only test that can "find that pain!" Unfortunately, unless there is a clear surgical alternative, once the pain source has been located, there is very little one can do to "cure" it.

The Electromyogram (EMG)

Then there is the EMG (electromyogram). Have you ever thought of yourself as a pincushion? Well, here's your chance. The EMG is carried out by someone trained in the procedure—usually a physician, but occasionally a physical therapist or a technician. It entails carefully placing fine needle electrodes into the muscles of your legs or back—a bit like acupuncture without the beneficial results. The electrodes measure the electricity that is transmitted to your muscles by the nerves to the muscles. The electrical pattern is then displayed on a TV tube. The tester takes a look at the "pictures" the electricity creates and can tell whether they show sick nerve roots from the spine, sick nerves in the legs, or sick muscles. Then, knowing the anatomy of the muscle he or she is testing, the tester can pinpoint where in your body the sick nerves reside. He or she can also tell, in general, how long the nerves have been sick and how severe the sickness is. These findings help your doctor diagnose your spinal condition.

Now, what can you do to help yourself get better, without a lot of prescription medicines, therapy, or surgery? Read on to find out.

EVERYDAY LIFE TREATMENTS

There are a few things that you can do, and control, in your everyday life that will help you maintain a healthy back. First of all, don't allow yourself to get "out of shape." That doesn't mean that you have to train like a pentathlon athlete. Just try to stay in some semblance of good physical condition. Remember that each extra pound that you add to your body weight has to be borne every day, 365 days a year, for perhaps 85 years, by the discs or shock absorbers of the low back. Very few low backs can stand up to this added load over this length of time without rebelling—causing pain! In fact, 80 percent of us will suffer some significant low back pain in our lives, even if we are pentathlon athletes. So watch your weight! And don't just watch it go higher and higher! Eat right! And if you don't know how to eat right, or what it means to eat right, get some help. Ask your doctor or a nutritionist to help you. It may cost you a few bucks, but it will save a great deal more in painful lost time from work or in medical bills for treatment of a painful back. (Or you could simply read Chapter 13.)

Exercise

Next, exercise! I know, I know, you hate to exercise. It's boring, it's expensive (all those fancy clothes and health-club bills), and it hurts! But you don't have to get all dressed up, check in, and do the same thing for an hour. Just walk more often! Climb up and down the steps instead of waiting for the elevator all the time. Ride your bicycle to the corner store instead of driving your car.

If you decide to purchase a treadmill for home use, or if you do join a health club and get some advice from one of those great-looking "therapists," well, more power to you. You're doing yourself and your low back a great favor.

Now you say, exercise sounds like it's good for me—good for my heart, good for my arteries—but what does it have to do with my low back? A treadmill can't give me stronger bones, or stronger discs, can it? No, it can't! But it can strengthen your back and abdominal muscles, and they protect your back from being injured by excess loading of those bones and discs by activities such as repetitive bending from the waist, lifting, twisting, and straining. We'll talk more about these activities later, but for now just realize that these are activities that you do every day that actually endanger the health of your low back. So, if your back and abdominal muscles are in reasonably good condition, you can prevent injury from these so-called normal activities of daily living.

Okay, now you're eating well, maintaining a healthy weight, and you're exercising. Is that all there is to maintaining a healthy back? Noooooo! Not by a long shot. If you really want to preserve your back, consider how you sleep, how you stand, how you sit, how you bend, how you lift and carry, how you twist, and how you drive.

How You Sleep

How you sleep really refers to what you sleep on. The firmer the surface the better. An extra-firm mattress with a ¾-inch plywood board underneath is the optimum surface. Soft mattresses and sofas allow the spine to "sag." This sagging distorts the discs or shock absorbers in the spine, and over time (overnight, in fact) this distortion can cause pain. That's why when you get up in the morning from sleeping on your sofa (temporarily) you have a stiff and sore back.

How You Stand

How you stand refers to your posture and the length of time you are standing. If you are standing in line at Disney World with your child, you may be there a long time. So keep moving. Since you certainly can't move forward, move sideways: shift your weight from one foot to the other. Anything that keeps those discs active as shock absorbers is good. You know what happens when shocks "bottom out"—you're in for a bumpy (read "painful") ride. Lean on something—a post, a fence, your four-year-old—anything that can temporarily unload those discs. Now about your posture. The worst thing you can do is relax. When you relax, your belly sticks out in front and your butt sticks out in back, causing an abnormal curvature of the spine known as a hyperlordosis or swayback. This position puts the greatest stress on the discs of the lower spine—and stress on the disc for any length of time hurts! So suck in that gut and tuck in that tail.

Sitting

Learn how to sit properly. "You're kidding!" you say. "I've been sitting all my life. It's not rocket science!" No it's not, but there is a proper and an improper way to sit as far as good spinal health is concerned. For example, just as you shouldn't sleep on the soft sofa, you shouldn't sit in a soft chair for any length of time. It offers no support to your spine. Your muscles will fatigue trying to support your spine, and your back will begin to hurt after a period of time. Does that mean that you can never sit on Grandma's sofa? No, of course not. But don't sit there too long! The best chair is one that completely and firmly supports your spine in a flexed or bent position. The worse type of chair pokes you in the back, and makes you sit in a hyperlordotic position, like a secretary's typing chair. And remember those of us with "mature" spines should never sit too long in any chair without getting up and moving about—to get those shock absorbers pumped up again. And if the chairman of the board tells you to sit down, inform him that you are just maintaining a healthy spine—"The better to work harder for you, sir!"

Don't Bend Over

Don't bend over! Never? Well, hardly ever. Of all body movements, bending from the waist puts the greatest stress on the low back discs (except straightening up from a bent position with a seventy-five-pound valise gripped tightly in your hands). It has to do with biomechanics, forces placed on our bodies by certain loads (the weight of our trunk multiplied by the distance of the center of our trunk back to our spine). Well, how do you pick up your slippers, the newspaper, or the paper clip that falls on the floor? Bend your knees! How about tying your shoes? Put one foot up on a bench or a chair. Address "little people" by squatting down to their level. Get use to it, and you will save yourself a great deal of spinal grief.

Lifting

Everyone has to lift things, don't they? Yes, of course. We carry packages home from the grocery store, we carry books at school, we carry briefcases to work, and we carry luggage on vacation. But there are proper and improper ways to lift and carry as far as spinal health is concerned. In the first place, never lift any object that is too heavy for you! That sounds dumb (how on earth are you supposed to know what weight is too heavy?), but it's a good general rule. Don't pack those grocery bags to the top. Use two bags. Pack fewer bottles and books into your vacation bag. If you can control the loads that you lift, make sure that they are as light as possible. What if you can't control the load? You have to lift Grandma's 150-pound trunk into your car. Well, get help—don't be macho—your spine doesn't know from macho! Also, don't lift from the floor by bending over. Bend your knees!

There is also a right and a wrong way to carry objects as far as spinal health is concerned. The closer the load is to your body, the better it is for your back. Backpacks are good. Carrying rocks in a shovel is bad!

Twisting

The next subject is the twist—not the dance, but the action of twisting our trunks while standing still. Lumbar discs don't handle twisting well. In fact, the only thing more detrimental to the discs than twisting is twisting with a load or weight in our hands. I'll only say this once—shoveling snow (or coal), moving rocks, and transferring books from a bookshelf are bad for the spine. And golf? Well, that's good healthy exercise—isn't it? Young, healthy discs in well-muscled individuals can get away (most of the time) with activities that require twisting. Do you fit in this category? If not, 'nuff said.

Driving

And now to driving. Car seats are not designed to maintain the health of your spine. They are meant to keep you as comfortable as possible while you drive or ride in a car. No matter how comfortable you are, driving is still hard on your back. So don't drive too far for your back. Drive for an hour or two, then take a stand-up break (after you stop the car, of course). Newer, more expensive cars do have a number of "back-saving mechanisms." Use them, of course, but getting out of the driver's seat (or the passenger seat) is still healthier for your back than staying in it for hours at a time.

There, that should give you a few important things to think about. More important, it should give you the power to help yourself get better and back into a more normal life.

COMPLIANCE AND ATTITUDE

Two final thoughts about "What can I do about it?" Let us examine the concepts of compliance and attitude. Compliance means doing what you are supposed to do—according to your health-care provider. The best medicine will not help if you don't take it. Attitude refers to the fact that you have to want to get better. You have to have hope for a treatment program to have a chance of helping you. If you are upbeat and adopt an optimistic attitude as you enter a program, you will have a better chance of improving your post-traumatic condition.

SUGGESTED READINGS

Dreyer, S.J., Boden, S.D. "Non Operative Treatment of Neck and Arm Pain," *Spine* 1998; 23:24, 2746–54.

Ernst, E. "The Role of Complementary and Alternative Medicine," *British Medical Journal* 2000; 321:1133–1135.

Horn, C. "Consumer Guide—13 Ways to Wipe Out Pain," *Natural Health,* Jan–Feb 1999; pp. 123–139.

Rose, M.J., et al. "Chronic Low Back Pain Rehabilitation Programs," *Spine,* 1997; 22:19, 2246–53.

HELPFUL WEB SITES

American Academy of Orthopaedic Surgeons
http://www.aaos.org

Healthfinder
http://www.healthfinder.gov

Medscape
http://www.medscape.com

Money Magazine
http://www.money.com/money/magazine/health/search.html

8

Prescriptions to Treat Chronic Pain

George E. Ehrlich, M.D.

Although everyone has pain, chronic pain that lasts for three months or more is an intensely personal experience. We feel this pain in varying degrees, and we express it and react to it in many different ways. For this reason, the treatment of chronic pain must be highly individual.

All of us have this much in common: Our perception of pain is always mental, even though the causes of pain may be located in other parts of the body, in the nerve endings or in the nerves themselves. Our bodies secrete substances at the sites of pain, including the mysterious substance P, which enhances the feeling of pain. Our bodies also produce prostaglandins, hormonelike substances that form at the site of an injury to energize the body's reparative responses. Prostaglandins also are present in various forms in other parts of the body where they have specific functions, either to combat injury and damage or to preserve the function of certain tissues and organs. Other substances also play a role in our perception of pain, and some may not as yet even have been discovered; this field of research is still evolving. However, many treatments for pain are designed to interact with substance P or prostaglandins.

EXERCISE—THE BEST PRESCRIPTION

It may surprise you to know that the most important treatment for chronic pain is exercise. The first precept in treating pain is to stay healthy, and keeping fit is all-important. Exercises that tone the body can prevent some painful states and can help control others. Leave bodybuilding to the professional athletes; often it's enough to walk instead of taking the car, breathe deeply, and do sit-ups, sit-downs (in which you sit on the floor, legs supported, and lean halfway back and then sit up again), and simple aerobics. These even help once pain has set in.

In response to exercise, the brain produces endorphins, and these chemicals block pain. Endorphins make it possible for athletes to run marathons, swim competitively, and lift extraordinary weights, because they dull the natural pain response. Any form of exercise energizes the production of endorphins and thus helps to control pain.

You may think that you can't exercise because you have pain. But no matter how much pain or fatigue you may experience, you can do some degree of exercise, and gradually more, so that you can bring your pain under control. You may need the help of a physical therapist to learn which exercises are best for you, how to tolerate them, and how to avoid making your problem worse. But just to keep moving will go a long way to helping you get over your pain.

It's also important to keep your weight down. Excess weight may not cause your pain, but it aggravates it by giving your body an additional burden to carry. You may feel that your pain keeps you inactive, and dieting is even more difficult if you sit around. Moving about and exercising prevent you from gaining unwanted weight. This doesn't mean that you have to give up your favorite foods or drinks; after all, everyone needs some joy in life, and for many people, meals and their accompaniment are part of that joy. But moderation is the key, as it has been since ancient times.

Closely related to your physical fitness is the size of your life space—that is, where you are able to go. If you remain shut in, then your room is your life space. If you are able to go out, how far do you go, and for what reasons? Can you go out to see your doctor; take a trip to the drugstore, the market, or the movies; or go to visit friends or relatives? Do you walk haltingly or briskly, or do you need to ride? Can you travel by car, or do you need transportation for the disabled? The size of your life space affects how well you are able to care for yourself, how you perceive yourself, and how others perceive you. It also determines whether you will lead a lonely life that encourages you to brood and feel sorry for yourself, or whether you can lose yourself in pleasant diversions by socializing with family and friends. For many people, religion provides an additional shield against chronic pain; having faith that you can feel better is a powerful medicine.

All these factors—your physical fitness, your weight, and your life space—are measures of your quality of life, and each one of them is important in preventing, treating, and controlling pain.

PAIN RELIEVERS

Only you know how much pain you have and how much you are willing to bear. Many of us assess our pain and decide that we can tolerate it up to a certain level. When we exceed that level, we often resort to over-the-counter medicines, that is, medicines for which no prescription is needed. Usually, these are pain relievers, or analgesics. If you need to take any nonprescription medicine for more than ten days or so, you should consult a physician.

The most popular analgesic is acetaminophen, which is sold under many trade names, the best known of which is Tylenol. Nonaspirin Anacin and store brands that carry the word "acetaminophen" in small letters all amount to the same thing. Check the dosage; just because you don't need a prescription doesn't mean that you can be reckless. Like all medicines, too much is potentially harmful, so follow the directions carefully. Acetaminophen isn't entirely safe for everyone. You should not take it within a few hours of drinking any alcoholic beverage, and it can damage your liver if you are elderly or alcoholic.

Acetaminophen has largely supplanted aspirin as a pain reliever. Aspirin has been available since the end of the nineteenth century and was long considered the best and safest painkiller. Today, many people take very modest doses to prevent blood from clotting in their coronary arteries. As you can imagine, if aspirin effectively blocks clotting, it is not entirely safe. Its effect upon the stomach lining is often troublesome and can lead to ulcers and bleeding. In some instances, aspirin can trigger a severe allergic reaction that can be fatal if untreated. In children, a severe disease, Reye's syndrome, may occur when fevers are treated with aspirin.

It's a truism that any medication that is effective may, in some instances, produce some unwanted secondary effects, or side effects. These aren't common, but that's why you should read the labels and be aware of possible unwanted consequences and know how to deal with them.

Anti-Inflammatories

Aspirin, unlike acetaminophen, also treats inflammation. If you scald yourself or suffer a sunburn, the afflicted area becomes red, warm, painful, and swollen. That's the way that inflammation was defined for centuries. In the past quarter century, the molecular causes of these symptoms were discovered, and new drugs were developed to reduce inflammation.

Inflammation may underlie some chronic pain syndromes (although it probably plays no role in so-called fibromyalgia and chronic fatigue syndrome), so medicines that control inflammation may be prescribed to treat your pain. These include the nonsteroidal anti-inflammatory drugs (NSAIDs). These drugs contain no cortisone or other steroids, but they may relieve pain as effectively as cortisone and its derivatives, without its hormonal effects. The newer NSAIDs all have been prescribed to reduce inflammation and to reduce pain.

Inflammation control generally requires a prescription-strength dosage. In prescription strength, NSAIDs include many generic names, the most popular of which have been indomethacin, one of the oldest (marketed as Indocin); ibuprofen (Motrin); naproxen (Naprosyn); diclofenac (Voltaren); and many more, including tolmetin, nabumetone, sulindac, etodolac, oxaprozine, piroxicam, and ketoprofen.

As the patents on these drugs expire, other companies in addition to the original manufacturers make or sell them under a variety of new trade names. Often these companies also manufacture these drugs in smaller doses, at nonprescription strength, and market them as pain relievers. For example, ibuprofen has become commercially successful in its lower strength under names such as Advil and Nuprin, and naproxen is available without prescription as Aleve. Ketoprofen also is sold as an over-the-counter painkiller. You may have seen commercials in which an achy, pain-ridden older person takes one of these and becomes sprightly and

MEDICINES THAT RELIEVE PAIN (ANALGESICS)

Nonprescription (called over-the-counter and available in supermarkets, drugstores, and large markets) USA

Medication	Trade Name
Acetaminophen	Tylenol, nonaspirin pain reliever
Aspirin	Many brands
Ibuprofen	Advil, Nuprin, Motrin IB
Ketoprofen	Orudis KT, Actron
Naproxen sodium	Aleve

Prescription (pharmacies only, requiring doctor's prescription)
Relieve pain and reduce inflammation USA

Salicylates (related to aspirin, without acetylation)	
Choline magnesium trisalicylate	Trilisate
Choline salicylate	Arthropan
Magnesium salicylate	Magan
Salsalate	Disalcid

Nonsteroidal anti-inflammatory drugs (NSAIDs) prescription only USA	
Celecoxib	Celebrex (a specific COX-2 inhibitor)
Diclofenac sodium with misoprostil	Voltaren, Voltaren XR Arthrotec
Etodolac	Lodine, Lodine XL
Fenoprofen calcium	Nalfon
Flurbiprofen	Ansaid
Ibuprofen	Motrin
Indomethacin	Indocin, Indocin SR
Ketoprofen	Orudis, Oravail
Meclofenamate sodium	Meclomen
Meloxicam	Mobic
Nabumetone	Relafen
Naproxen	Naprosyn, Naprelan
Oxaprozine	Daypro
Piroxicam	Feldene
Rofecoxib	Vioxx (a specific COX-2 inhibitor)
Sulindac	Clinoril
Tolmetin sodium	Tolectin
Valdecoxib	Bextra

MEDICINES THAT RELIEVE PAIN (ANALGESICS) (cont'd)	
NSAIDs for pain relief (not or only mildly anti-inflammatory)	
Diclofenac potassium	Cataflam
Diflunisal	Dolobid
Mefenamic acid	Ponstel
Naproxen sodium	Anaprox
Topical pain relievers	
Capsaicin	Zostrix, many other trade names
Counter-irritants	Many different brands
Salicylates	Aspercreme, Ben Gay, many others

spry and happily capable of playing with his or her grandchildren. These may well be exaggerated claims, but these drugs can certainly suppress pain to some degree.

In recent years, the effects of these drugs upon prostaglandins have become better understood. The nonsteroidal anti-inflammatory drugs have a dual effect on prostaglandins: They inhibit those that are responsible for pain and inflammation, but they also inhibit those that protect the stomach lining, kidneys, membranes around the brain, and other organs. So NSAIDs do cause some unwanted effects—not in most people, but in some. That's why they are prescription drugs, because some monitoring—watching for signs of their effectiveness as well as their potential side effects—is necessary.

More recently, NSAIDs that chiefly inhibit only those prostaglandins that produce pain and inflammation have been developed. Several are still undergoing testing, but the ones that are available by prescription include celecoxib (Celebrex), rofecoxib (Vioxx), and valdecoxib (Bextra). The former is taken twice daily, the latter two once daily. While they seem to cause fewer stomach problems than older NSAIDs, they may still have an adverse effect upon other organs. For this reason, the federal Food and Drug Administration (FDA) gives them a class label, a label shared by all drugs in the same category, even though the risks or benefits may not be equal for all. Unfortunately for most sufferers of chronic pain, especially for those diagnosed with fibromyalgia and chronic fatigue syndrome, these drugs are only moderately effective, if at all.

None of these medicines should be expected to work quickly, and none will provide a cure. But together with a physical conditioning program and other nonmedical features, some among them might help to reduce the severity of your pain. The best advice is not to believe all the claims sent over the Internet and to be skeptical about any unusual treatments that might be advocated, especially by nonphysicians.

Analgesic Ointments

Some analgesics are available in the form of ointments that are sold without a prescription. These work best on very localized pains. After all, you can't really smear them all over your pain-ridden body several times a day, nor is that advisable. You may have seen commercials and advertisements for these products; by and large, they are meant for localized, acute pains, not for chronic pain. Many analgesics are available as creams and ointments in other countries, but most have not yet been approved in the United States. Most are classified as cosmetics by the FDA, which should tell you what this government watchdog agency thinks of their efficacy! An exception is capsaicin, the substance that makes chili peppers hot.

Capsaicin is available under a number of different names, both as a prescription and as a nonprescription ointment. Regular application over some joints afflicted with osteoarthritis or some areas of tenderness, such as tennis elbow or bursitis, gradually eliminates the painful effects of substance P. At first, it may burn, so you must be patient for several applications, and give it at least a week or more before you expect to feel relief. Be very careful to wash your hands thoroughly after applying it, as it would burn horribly if you were to get some in your eyes, or the mucous membranes of your mouth, or in any genital or gastrointestinal orifice. And as you cannot (or should not) smear it all over your body, especially repeatedly, it really is not an appropriate treatment for diffuse chronic pain.

Narcotics

Are there medicines that can get rid of your pain? Certainly you can obtain transient relief from narcotic medicines such as opiates. Codeine, acetaminophen with codeine, oxycodone (OxyContin), methadone, Tramadol, Fiorinal, and the fentanyl pain patches are the most popular. For a long time, physicians hesitated to prescribe these because of the possibility of addiction, but their judicious use under strict supervision, usually in hospital settings, is now generally considered appropriate. But the threat of habituation or addiction remains, and in the long run, these narcotics do not alter the course of chronic pain. These do not cure chronic pain; they only suppress it.

What can these painkillers accomplish? They can reduce your level of pain to one you can tolerate, but they probably will not completely remove chronic pain. Of course, they work fairly well for an ordinary headache or toothache. But chronic pain is different. A cycle of irritation and response has been set up in your body, and most painkillers cannot do more than briefly interrupt it.

Experimental Medications

In the hope of finding more effective treatments, other, more unusual drugs have recently been tried. You may have read about some of these in magazine or newspaper features that hail them as cures (although you never see a follow-up story reporting that many of the trumpeted treatments fail). One example is botulinum toxin, or Botox. Botulism is caused by a bacterium (*Clostridium*) that produces a muscle-paralyzing substance; the disease was named because it was found to be contracted by eating tainted sausages (*botulus* means "sausage") or food that had been imperfectly sealed in cans or bottles. The poison is now used medicinally by injecting small doses into the body to cause selective weakening and paralysis of muscles in an attempt to alleviate cramps, spasms, and pain. You may have read about this on the Internet as a "miracle cure" for fibromyalgia. Because Botox is a paralytic agent, prolonged use or overdose can produce serious side effects. As of now, there is no evidence that it really helps chronic pain; it certainly is not a cure, and it is very expensive.

Other medicines that have been used to treat chronic pain include immunoglobulins (on the theory that enhancing your immunity permits you to overcome the malady), alpha-globulins, Ampligen, terfenadine (an antihistamine), alpha-interferon, and staphylococcus toxoid, all presumably recommended on the same principle. None has been carefully studied as to its usefulness in treating chronic pain, and favorable results are difficult to substantiate; however, adverse side effects are common.

A host of other pharmacological interventions also have been reported, again with unverifiable benefit. Among these are derivatives of cortisone, such as hydrocortisone and fludrocortisone. An antiviral drug, acyclovir, has been given on the mistaken assumption that Epstein-Barr virus or some other virus might be responsible for the symptoms of chronic pain and fatigue.

Other drugs include moclobemide, fluoxetine, phenelzine, sibutramine, galanthamine hydrobromide, and selegiline. These generic drugs are sold under a number of trade names, but not one of them works to relieve chronic pain. Growth hormone has its advocates, but there is no proof of its usefulness in treating chronic pain, and there is considerable evidence of its potential harm.

COGNITIVE THERAPY

One particularly effective approach to chronic pain is cognitive therapy, at least according to some studies (although a recent reputable medical trial failed to show more than a modest benefit). This psychiatric technique, pioneered chiefly by Dr. Aaron Beck of Philadelphia, is a relatively short treatment of a period of weeks and explores the patient's psychological and social surroundings as well as physical symptoms. This approach appears to have produced excellent results in most of those who have availed themselves of it. But, like many forms of psychiatric intervention, a full course of treatment tends to be expensive.

Together with exercise and conditioning programs, cognitive therapy can reduce the distress of chronic pain to tolerable levels and, in some cases, can even subdue it entirely. Do not rule out cognitive therapy just because it is a form of psychiatry. To consider the role of the mind in the cause, duration, and control of pain is only appropriate; after all, that's where our perception of pain resides.

A GOOD NIGHT'S SLEEP

Some researchers believe that sleep disturbances may aggravate, and even cause, pain. This subject is controversial, because some well-controlled recent studies have cast doubt on sleep abnormalities as the cause of pain. However, pain may *result* in non-restful sleep. Sleeping pills aren't the answer, because they do little for the specific sleep disturbances that interfere with non-REM sleep, the deep, restorative sleep we all need.

Strangely, medicines used by psychiatrists to relieve depression and elevate mood actually work better than sleeping pills to restore proper sleep. A small dose—less than the psychiatric dose—taken within half an hour of bedtime helps restore the deep-sleep phases and lets you feel more rested; as a result, this reduces the amount of pain you experience. Amitriptyline (Elavil) and Paxil have been used for this purpose. So have some antiepileptic medicines, such as Neurontin and Tegretol, which affect the central nervous system in ways that help to interrupt the pain cycle. Prozac also has been used, with indifferent results.

STRESS MANAGEMENT

Stress inevitably makes your pain worse. Impending stress such as a visit to the doctor or preparing for company will increase your symptoms. Be aware of this, and get in the habit of breathing deeply and learning stress-avoidance techniques so that your pain will not be punctuated by worse pain. The slogan "Don't worry, be happy" will give you the right message if only you can avail yourself of it.

You can derive some benefits from massages, saunas, whirlpools, and from soaking in warm (but never hot) baths—but always in conjunction with the effective treatments mentioned above. What all these therapies have in common is relaxation, which loosens tight muscles. But once again, these are not cures, even though they may be effective treatments, at least in the short term.

ALTERNATIVE TREATMENTS

Elsewhere in this book you will read about alternative treatments for chronic pain. Health-food supplements and vitamins often are recommended, although usually not by physicians. They have become big business, despite the fact that their effectiveness for pain control remains to be proved. The health foods and other supplements most often favored include essential fatty acids, magnesium, liver extract, and a host of general supplements; none has proved helpful. In a way, the large sums of money spent on these products are testimony that people aren't fully satisfied with the medicines that are available, even by prescription.

Interestingly, many people don't regard these products as medicines, although they are (even though Congress currently exempts them from FDA control). Many people take these natural products in addition to what their doctors order, and see no problem. But there might well be a problem, because some of these products interact with medicines prescribed for a number of conditions and diseases, perhaps to the detriment of both: The effectiveness of medicine may be reduced, or a serious side effect may result from the interaction. If you take any of these products, be sure to report what you are taking to your physician so that this can be taken into account when medicines are prescribed.

Yoga has been found to help relieve chronic pain, particularly in India and other southern Asian areas, and its recent popularity in the United States has demonstrated how helpful it is to many a sufferer who learns its techniques. Acupuncture, too, has been touted and may offer relief if done by an expert and with a receptive group, at least for localized pains. However, much of what is accomplished with acupuncture in China has yet to be duplicated on a large scale in the West.

Chiropractic adjustment is popular and can bring some relief from pain if there are no physical restrictions or contraindications. Some studies show that patients prefer it to drug therapy, but it generally costs more in time and money, and not everyone is convinced of its effectiveness. Osteopathic physicians used to learn to manipulate the body, which is similar to chiropractic adjustment; in fact, their discipline was founded on manipulation. However, in later years, many osteopaths have not been trained in manipulation.

CLINICS

Pain management has become a specialty, and you can find pain clinics at hospitals and at other locations in most cities. Avoid so-called fibromyalgia clinics and treatment centers. Many health professionals staff these, but their so-called multidisciplinary treatments have yet to be shown to have validity or to successfully ameliorate the symptoms over time.

Some people travel to Tijuana or other Mexican border clinics, some of which advertise extensively, especially on the Internet. Avoid these clinics; they can't help you, but they may harm you. The medicines they sell are usually mixtures of products, many of which the FDA has either refused to approve or regulates scrupulously. You lose this protection when you take drugs offered by a border clinic, and you risk serious, even fatal, side effects.

CLIMATE

Many of those who can afford it seek out warm climates in the hope of achieving relief. Consistent weather, though not necessarily warm weather, seems to work best. Every change of weather seems to bring on symptoms, and it's not a superstition that sufferers from chronic pain can predict weather changes. But the proportion of people who have the symptoms associated with what some call fibromyalgia and chronic fatigue syndrome is the same in the warm areas of the Gulf Coast and the Southwest as it is in Boston, Minneapolis, and Portland.

YOU MAY NOT be able to escape chronic pain, but you can avoid falling into the trap of chronic invalidism. The trauma you sustained that you blame for your pains probably only drew them to your attention and was unlikely the cause. Avoid falling into the trap of patient-advocacy groups that seek to persuade you that you can't get well. Don't let anyone talk you into chronic illness. You can—and you will—get better. Generally, no treatment is given in isolation, so a combination of drugs and physical approaches is usually best.

Live your life and think positively. Keep up your conditioning program, consider cognitive therapy, and avoid unnecessary tests and treatments. Most important, realize that pain is a human condition that we all experience and one that you need not completely abolish to function normally and enjoy life.

SUGGESTED READING

Arthritis Today

A magazine published by the Arthritis Foundation.

9

Treating Your Symptoms after a Concussion

ARNOLD SADWIN, M.D.

The physical and emotional pain caused by a head injury can be treated in many ways. Some symptoms of post-concussion syndrome (PCS) may persist for weeks or months, and some may even be permanent. However, most of these injuries can be treated, and many of them will diminish or disappear in time.

In this chapter, you'll find out how to cope with the forty most common symptoms of PCS, with information about medication, psychotherapy, and other treatments. Of course, as with any injury, be sure to consult your personal physician if you experience any of these symptoms.

HEADACHES

Headaches are among the most common problems that result from a closed-head injury, so common that they occur in 95 percent of our patients. However, they also are among the most difficult problems to treat.

After a concussion, headaches may be constant and severe, and they may not respond to over-the-counter medication. Your doctor may have to prescribe narcotics such as Percocet, OxyContin, or Demerol until the pain begins to lessen and becomes intermittent. This may take several weeks. At that time, the pain may respond to less restricted prescribed medications such as Fiorinal, Fioricet, or Midrin. Tylenol with codeine also can be helpful. As the pain subsides even further, over-the-counter medications may suffice, including Tylenol, aspirin, or Excedrin.

Be careful not to take more medication than you need in order to prevent rebound headaches, which can be caused by the frequent use of any of these pain medicines. Of course, you also should keep your physician advised of the frequency and severity of your headaches. Keeping a record of your headaches on a graph will help you and your doctor to observe the frequency of your headaches, your response to various medications, and your gradual improvement.

Because migraine headaches can be triggered by a closed-head injury or can be reactivated even if you have not had a headache for years, it is wise to talk to a neurologist or a family doctor who is trained to treat this problem with the specialized medications that can be prescribed. These include nasal sprays, self-administered injections, or pills to swallow or to place under your tongue. Each of these medications has side effects that you will need to discuss with your doctor, and their use should be carefully supervised by him or her. If you have heart problems, you will need to be extra careful about using these migraine medications.

An injury in which the back of the head has been struck by a headrest or another object can cause pain in the back of the head, where the occipital nerves are located. This condition is known as occipital neuralgia and is not difficult to diagnose. It causes the back of the head to be very tender, but injections of Marcaine or Carbocaine to block the occipital nerves bring rapid relief that may last for hours, days, weeks, or months. Then additional injections can be given at increasing intervals of time.

Many alternative treatments are available for headaches and are discussed in other chapters, including acupuncture, biofeedback, cognitive behavioral therapy, nutritional supplements, hypnosis, and the use of electric stimulators.

One electronic gadget that can reduce headache pain as well as the need for medication is the Alpha-Stim 100. This handheld device is about the size of a TV remote and conveys a mild electric current to the head through leads that clip on to the earlobes. The current can be reg-

TREATMENTS FOR HEADACHE PAIN

- Medication.
- Acupuncture.
- Biofeedback.
- Electric stimulation.
- Nutritional supplements.
- Individual or group therapy.
- Cognitive behavioral therapy.
- Hypnosis.

ulated to a level that causes you to feel no more than a slight tingling. The unit has a timer that usually is set at twenty minutes, and treatment can be repeated during the day. The unit is lightweight, so it can be easily carried.

Another handheld electronic device is the Solitens unit, which is used to apply an electrical pulse to tense muscles. By relaxing muscle spasms in the neck, this may alleviate some headache pain. This unit also can be easily carried and used repeatedly, but be sure not to use it near your eyes or the carotid arteries in your neck.

Head pain that is caused by damage to the jaw should be evaluated and treated by a dental specialist. Sometimes physical therapy or the use of a prosthesis is helpful. It's a good idea to talk over this problem with your dentist so that you have a better understanding of how this injury may be a cause of headaches.

Since headaches are so common and so difficult to treat, all pain therapies are worth trying until one is successful.

NAUSEA AND VOMITING

Nausea and vomiting usually subside during the first few weeks following a concussion. They do not necessarily need any special treatment (unless they occur just after an accident, at which time the possibility of brain swelling requires careful neurologic examination). Sometimes this problem improves when headaches improve. In extreme cases, Compazine or Tigan suppositories may help.

BLURRED VISION

Blurred vision is one of the first symptoms to subside after a concussion. However, you might need to have your eyes examined, and you shouldn't be surprised if you are told for the first time that you need reading glasses; if you already have them, you may need stronger lenses.

DOUBLE VISION

Double vision needs to be evaluated by a neuro-ophthalmologist if it remains constant after an accident or continues to recur intermittently for several weeks. If you're lucky, it may subside without treatment.

SENSITIVITY TO BRIGHT LIGHTS

Sensitivity to bright lights is best dealt with by wearing glasses with tinted lenses. This problem may persist indefinitely.

DIFFICULTY HEARING

Difficulty hearing must be evaluated by an otologist (an ear doctor), who can determine whether you need a hearing aid.

SENSITIVITY TO LOUD NOISES

Sensitivity to loud noises should subside almost as quickly as blurred vision. In the meantime, try using earplugs, turning down the volume, asking people to lower their voices, or avoiding sources of loud noise.

RINGING IN YOUR EARS

Ringing in your ears is an annoyance that probably will disappear eventually, providing that it's not constant. If it persists constantly, there isn't much that can be done, but if you discuss it with an otologist (an ear doctor), you may find a device that can override the ringing. Alternatively, you might be able to adjust to it.

DIZZINESS

Dizziness is a spinning sensation that may occur when you move your head, get up from a chair, or when you get out of bed too quickly. This is more likely to be a problem if your inner ear has suffered a concussion. Medications such as Antivert are often prescribed for this condition, but they may make you sleepy. If this problem persists, see an ear, nose, and throat specialist.

LIGHT-HEADEDNESS

Light-headedness may make you feel faint. If you occasionally feel that you may lose consciousness—or if you black out—ask your doctor to check your blood pressure while you are lying down and then to recheck it after you stand up quickly. If your blood pressure drops significantly, you may benefit from the use of support hosiery. Until this problem improves, be careful to move your head slowly, and take your time when you move to a standing position.

SEIZURES

Seizures are quite serious, especially if they are not properly diagnosed and treated. Most of the time, an electroencephalogram (EEG) is not helpful as a diagnostic tool, unless it is a digital (quantitative) EEG, which has greater diagnostic value and is less likely to give a false-negative reading. However, a normal brain-wave tracing does not rule out the presence of a seizure disorder. Diagnosis is usually made from a patient's medical history, especially if a seizure has been witnessed by someone who can describe it to the doctor in minute detail. It is most helpful to keep a record of the frequency of your seizures to show to your doctor.

Anticonvulsive medication that is commonly prescribed includes Depakote, Tegretol, Dilantin, or Neurontin. Before taking any of these drugs, you should review their side effects with your doctor, and blood studies should be done during the course of treatment in order to maintain therapeutic blood levels. If you do not improve, your doctor probably will increase the dosage, combine more than one medication, or switch to a different medication altogether.

If you are having periods of unconsciousness, you must not drive. You also should avoid heights and should not work around moving machinery, swim alone, ride a bicycle, or use a ladder.

Seizures that occur after a head injury most often subside within a few years. But unless they are treated, they may result in repeated concussions.

DISORIENTATION

Episodes of disorientation, or spells, should be noted on a graph to be shown to your physician. This will help your physician to evaluate your condition and will help you to eliminate the anxiety that follows each episode. At present, no medication is available to remedy this problem, but it usually subsides on its own.

Talking about these spells, especially in group therapy, can be most helpful. If you feel disoriented, knowing that you are not the only one may reduce your fear. (See "Group Therapy" on page 150.)

PROBLEMS WITH BALANCE

Problems with balance may indicate an injury to your inner ear, so you should be evaluated by an otologist (an ear doctor). Sometimes medication such as Antivert can be helpful.

CLUMSINESS OR STAGGERING

Clumsiness or staggering, like other problems with balance, requires you to pay special attention so that you do not bump into things and sustain another concussion. Unfortunately, this happens all too often. Physical therapy may help you to re-coordinate your body movements, and you may need gait retraining. Discuss this with your physician and physical therapist. In the meantime, remove potentially dangerous obstacles such as slippery throw rugs from your home and office, and make a mental note of hazards such as overhanging cabinets or Dutch doors.

ERRORS IN DEPTH PERCEPTION

Errors in depth perception and the impairment of your keen awareness of your surroundings will require that you pay much more attention to your environment. Make a note of potential objects that might put you in harm's way. Watch out for curled rugs, protruding cabinets, sharp corners, narrow passageways, door frames, rocks on the ground, steep steps, and other objects that might require a careful assessment of potential risk.

CHANGE IN HANDWRITING

A change in handwriting often improves in time without treatment. In the meantime, there is not much to do about it except to practice writing more slowly and perhaps revert to printing.

CHANGES IN COLOR PERCEPTION

Changes in color perception, such as distinguishing navy blue from black, require you to make some adjustments. Little can be done except to acknowledge the situation and to ask others to help you if necessary. This condition may be permanent.

CHANGES IN TASTE OR SMELL

Changes in taste or smell may be permanent, especially if you experience a complete loss of either sense. When you are away from home, you should take extra precautions to protect yourself with a portable smoke detector. Your family and friends should understand why you have changed your choices in food or the way you now use seasoning. When you cook for others, you may want to ask them to add more of their own flavoring.

LOSS OF APPETITE

Loss of appetite can be part of post-concussion syndrome, but it also can be a symptom of hidden depression. Your doctor should make sure you have not developed other medical problems. If nothing else can explain your loss of appetite, then get yourself evaluated for a mood disorder, because you may be in need of an antidepressant.

INCREASED APPETITE

Increased appetite may be caused by anxiety and/or depression. Now is the time to be more consciously aware of sensible dieting. An increase in appetite also may be the side effect of some prescription medications.

JUNK FOOD CRAVINGS

A craving for junk food most often subsides, but until that happens, you can do something about it: Take one or two bites of whatever you are craving and follow it with two glasses of cold water. The water dilutes the food, speeding its absorption and transmitting nutrients to your brain more quickly. It also rinses your teeth and helps to prevent cavities, while at the same time it fills your stomach and reduces your immediate craving.

WEIGHT GAIN OR LOSS

A gain or loss of weight should be reported to your physician, and it's important to keep a record of your weight so that your doctor can determine the seriousness of any change. Gaining weight can become very depressing, especially if you continually gain and do nothing about it. You need all the help you can get, so talk with your doctor about this.

SLEEP DISTURBANCES

Sleep disturbance should be treated with the appropriate medication if you have trouble falling asleep or staying asleep. Taking 10 milligrams of Ambien, a sleeping pill, just before you turn out the lights can be helpful. If you are worried about becoming habituated to sleeping pills, take one every other night after the first two weeks of steady use. Then gradually reduce the frequency and dosage, or alternate it with other sleeping medication such as Halcion, ProSom, Sonata, Restoril, Placidyl, or chloral hydrate in capsule or liquid form.

Over-the-counter health-food products are sometimes used successfully. These products are not without risk, so be sure to inform your physician about them. Read about what you are using. Be aware of potential problems such as drug interactions, harmful side effects, and addictive potential. Keeping careful records of the dosage and frequency of every medication you use may help to avoid complications.

Sometimes, when physical pain interferes with sleep, the use of effective pain medication might take the place of a sleeping pill. Tranquilizers such as Xanax and Valium are occasionally prescribed to help an anxious patient fall asleep. In the meantime, eliminate caffeinated beverages, at least until your sleep pattern returns to normal.

NIGHTMARES

Nightmares are one method the brain uses to gradually expel some of the stored fear and rage activated by trauma. Nightmares may subside if intensive psychotherapy is used to help reduce the residual emotional disturbance caused by the accident. Sometimes hypnosis may be effective, too. Treatment of anxiety disorders also may help. Most patients find that this problem takes care of itself in due time.

DAYTIME FLASHBACKS

Daytime flashbacks gradually subside on their own, but treatment should help hasten the process. Individual and group psychotherapy usually helps. (See "Group Therapy" on page 150.)

TIREDNESS OR CHRONIC FATIGUE

Tiredness or chronic fatigue may improve if your sleep problems subside. However, fatigue is a common problem even among PCS patients who sleep excessively.

Currently we are prescribing Provigil, which is marketed primarily for patients with narcolepsy (brief attacks of sleep). We have found this to be useful in treating the daytime fatigue that is part of PCS. Taking 100–200 milligrams of Provigil once or twice a day can result in increased daytime energy, improved self-esteem, and a better sleep pattern.

IRRITABILITY

Irritability is a serious problem, especially when it reaches the level of a rage reaction. A brain injury may cause significant changes in personality and loss of self-control. Medications that should be tried include the various anticonvulsants such as Tegretol, Depakote, and Neurontin, in addition to minor and major tranquilizers best prescribed by a psychiatrist. A combination of medicine and psychotherapy, either individual or group, can help protect your marriage, your job, and your social life. Biofeedback is beneficial, too. (See "Biofeedback" on page 152.)

GROUP THERAPY

You may be angry with the person who was responsible for your injury—or, if the accident was your fault, you may be angry with yourself. You also may be disappointed in yourself for losing your "smarts" after suffering microscopic brain damage from head trauma. Talking about your mental discomfort with a therapist and in a group will enable you to vent your anguish and disappointment.

At first you might have difficulty finding a proper support group. Many are associated with head-injury foundations. Be sure the one you choose deals with so-called minor head injuries and post-concussion syndrome; otherwise you may not feel at home with the more seriously injured patients. You need to be able to identify with other folks who look fine but who have the same symptoms you developed after your concussion.

During the first session, you should try to explain how your accident happened and describe your post-concussion symptoms. Unlike at a party, where you may be likely to withdraw to the quiet part of the room, in a group you are sitting among new friends who will not overwhelm you with too much input. They know that multiple conversations can be confusing.

These groups should meet no less than once a week and are best limited to about eight post-concussion patients led by a trained psychotherapist. All members of the group should be able to discuss whatever symptoms are interfering with their happiness. They also should call attention to anything that is improving and share with the others whatever may have helped them get better.

You will soon be able to discuss the embarrassing mental injuries you probably have been trying to deny. By talking about your difficulties with others who share them, you will begin to learn how to deal with them and to be more accepting of yourself. Others will share with you some of the solutions they have found, their tricks of the trade.

Your treatment will be more successful if you are able to redirect your energy from feeling sorry for yourself to helping your brain to recover. Mental exercises such as doing daily crossword puzzles or playing along with trivia games on TV are the easiest to do. Memory games introduced at group therapy can be brought home to share with your family. The funnier the games, the better. Without laughter you are at a disadvantage. Finding something to laugh about in the face of mental and physical pain is therapeutic and even better if shared with others. This will lift your spirits and raise the level of everyone's endorphins, the pain-relieving chemicals that our bodies make.

This author has been holding weekly group meetings with post-concussion patients for nearly twenty years in Philadelphia, Pennsylvania, and nearby Cherry Hill, New Jersey. This has been a very helpful method of treatment that has enabled many patients to stay socially active and has hastened the rehabilitation of many of the 6,000 head-injury patients we have seen.

DIFFICULTY CONCENTRATING AND FOCUSING

Difficulty concentrating and focusing causes your mind to wander. You're easily distracted. You may find yourself rereading the same sentences or paragraphs over and over again. You may not comprehend what you are trying to read. You may even give up reading for pleasure. If so, you'll have to find new ways of doing old things; it's as if your autopilot is broken.

You may need the services of a cognitive remedial therapist who can teach practical techniques to those who have PCS. Working on a one-to-one basis, cognitive remedial therapists explain how to remove distractions, how to stay focused, and how to create and use schedules in order to remember appointments. They often make phone calls to check up on patients in addition to seeing patients at their offices.

If you are having great difficulty reading, you may have to go back to early basic readers like the ones you used in grammar school and gradually work your way up. If you do this, you will be pleasantly surprised at how your mind can "regrow." It may not be easy, but think of it as going back to stick-shifting instead of using an automatic gearshift. You should see slow but continual improvement.

BIOFEEDBACK

Biofeedback is a treatment method that makes it possible for you to observe your physical reactions to stress and pain, using electrical sensors that can detect minute changes in your body temperature, degree of sweating, and heart rate.

The first goal of biofeedback is to make you aware of the level of stress in your body. The information gathered by instruments that monitor your muscle tension, skin temperature, breathing, pulse, and perspiration is "fed back" to you in the form of a graph or as an audible tone, so that you can see your level of tension or hear it on a speaker.

Then you are taught techniques of muscle relaxation, abdominal breathing, the use of imagery, and verbal suggestion. These help you learn to take some conscious control over the part of your nervous system that is making you uncomfortable and is otherwise automatic. In order to be able to use this therapy, you should be treated two or three times a week by a biofeedback therapist and then practice these skills at home with relaxation tapes, using the monitors to observe the results.

This training cannot cure an injury, but most people experience a significant decrease in their perception of their pain. Learning how to gain more control over your body's reactions reduces your feelings of helplessness and discomfort. This should increase your response to other treatments and help improve your self-esteem.

DIFFICULTY REMEMBERING RECENT EVENTS

Difficulty remembering recent events can be eased by using techniques taught by cognitive remedial therapists. These methods include making lists, reminder notes, using alarm clocks and timers, keeping an extra set of keys, asking someone else to manage the checkbook, and sticking to a schedule. Doing crossword puzzles is good mental exercise to help repair the brain.

One medication that has been helpful in treating memory problems in patients with Alzheimer's disease is called Aricept. Some head-injury specialists have found that it also may help post-concussion patients. Medications used for attention-deficit disorders, such as Ritalin-SR, Concerta, or Adderall, are now being prescribed to help patients with PCS to improve their concentration, multi-tasking abilities, and mental focus.

DIFFICULTY FINDING WORDS

Difficulty finding words and expressing thoughts can be embarrassing, but carrying a pocket dictionary and explaining your problem to others may enable you to avoid frustration. Usually, in due time, word-finding problems and difficulty expressing your thoughts will subside.

DIFFICULTY FOLLOWING A SEQUENCE

Difficulty following a sequence can be alleviated in time with practice. A cognitive remedial therapist can suggest many helpful techniques.

Using a computer and a handheld calculator can help to reestablish mental efficiency. You may have to ask for a lot of help. This may be embarrassing, especially if you were good at using a computer before your head injury and then forgot how. Find a very patient, understanding friend who can retrain you and allow for ongoing forgetfulness for a while. Ask your friend to read this part of the book. Learn how to quit feeling foolish! With time and practice, you will improve.

Write down explicit directions and be extra careful when using road maps. Avoid any interference as you repeatedly review directions. If this is impractical, or if it remains a problem even without interference, you must ask others for assistance, and then, hopefully, you will still be able to work or attend school.

DIFFICULTY PERFORMING MULTIPLE TASKS

Difficulty performing multiple tasks may require the help of a cognitive remedial therapist. As previously mentioned, Ritalin-SR can help.

At home, ask your loved ones not to overburden you with questions when you are in the middle of trying to do something. They also should be aware that you could easily lose your temper if they interrupt when you are involved with even simple tasks.

It is wisest to do more complicated tasks when you have more energy, which is typically in the morning. Try to do things when others are not around to confuse you. Because you will tire more easily after a concussion, try not to burden yourself with more than basic responsibility later in the day.

DIFFICULTY UNDERSTANDING CONVERSATION

Difficulty understanding conversation should be dealt with at the time it happens by asking for clarification. Group therapy can be very helpful in enabling patients to overcome their embarrassment, because they have to admit their shortcomings in order for others to cooperate with them. In group therapy, it's easier to ask someone to slow down, repeat, or explain more clearly what they have to say. (See "Group Therapy" on page 150.)

ANXIETY, FEARS, AND PHOBIAS

Anxiety, fears, and phobias caused by trauma warrant individual and group therapy as well as biofeedback and the use of medications. Anxiety is commonly treated with Ativan, Librium, Tranxene, Valium, Xanax, or Vistaril. An acute attack can be treated with small amounts of Xanax, placed under the tongue. Antidepressants such as Celexa, Effexor, Prozac, Serzone, Paxil, and Zoloft also are useful. Anticonvulsants have been successfully used to treat some patients who suffer from panic attacks, especially those whose spells resemble seizures. (See "Group Therapy" on page 150 and "Biofeedback" on page 152.)

HALLUCINATIONS

Hallucinations usually are not serious. They usually do not require any more treatment than reassurance. Some doctors do not know that mistaken perceptions such as hearing your name being called or seeing bugs that are not there are often a temporary part of PCS and not outright psychosis. However, if you become paranoid, you will need psychiatric help.

Talking about your hallucinations, especially in group therapy, will give you significant mental relief once you find out that others have had these minor hallucinations. (See "Group Therapy" on page 150.)

DEPRESSION

Depression is best treated with a combination of medication and psychotherapy. Many antidepressant medicines can be tried, and you should become informed about their side effects. Medicine should be started at a low dose and gradually increased in an effort to minimize or avoid side effects. You may be more sensitive to side effects of medication just because you have had a concussion. (By the way, you also may be more sensitive to alcohol.) If an antidepressant does not help within three to six weeks, it is either the wrong medicine or the wrong dosage.

Psychotherapy, either individual or group, will help if you learn why you became depressed. Some of your depression may be alleviated when you discover that it is part of post-concussion syndrome, not early Alzheimer's disease. Ask your therapist to explain the relationship of your depression to your head injury. This should help relieve any guilt you may have developed when your depression appeared. If you had a previous depression that was successfully treated, you can look forward to similar improvement. Talking over the problems caused by the mental and emotional changes that occur after a concussion will lead to psychological relief.

One major cause of depression after an accident is the sudden loss of part of your identity. You may ask, "Where am I? Where did the real me go?" You may feel as if part of you has died. Depression is the mourning of your former self. Psychotherapy is directed toward helping you to understand what happened and then to use all the methods available to deal with each symptom.

One important warning: If suicidal thoughts occur, you must inform your doctor, so that appropriate treatment can be instituted immediately!

MENSTRUAL PROBLEMS

Persistent problems with the menstrual cycle should be treated by a gynecologist, but normality usually returns after a few months.

LOSS OF AMBITION

Loss of ambition is a symptom that may fade as headaches, fatigue, depression, and disturbed sleep are successfully treated. When you begin to feel a little better and are able to do more, your improved self-esteem helps to restore feelings of ambition.

LOSS OF LIBIDO

Loss of libido that is attributed to the concussion itself, and not associated with the side effects of any medication, requires individual or couples counseling. Impotence responds favorably to Viagra, but no medication has yet proven effective in helping women to overcome the loss of libido associated with PCS.

Discussing sexual impairment, either individually or as a couple, reduces feelings of guilt and rejection. It can save a relationship and stop emotional pain. Of course, it's more difficult to talk about this in group therapy than with a private counselor. Try to get over your embarrassment and talk about it; it should help.

LOSS OF SELF-ESTEEM

Loss of self-esteem may be somewhat restored as you get used to your symptoms and forgive yourself for losing part of yourself. You have to stop asking yourself, "Where am I, what happened to me, and when will I get better?" Wasting time bemoaning your partial loss of self takes away the energy you need to help recover as much as you can.

There is no way to know how long it will take for you to achieve whatever degree of improvement you are going to experience. Until then, group therapy is highly recommended to enable you to get past your anger, frustration, depression, and disappointment at losing part of yourself. (See "Group Therapy" on page 150.)

REMEMBER, there is usually some degree of recovery from almost any injury. Recovering from post-concussion syndrome should be a team effort engaging you, your family, your boss, your teachers, and all the therapists trained to put Humpty Dumpty back together again. Group therapy is among the best methods, because it places you among friends who are going through the same problems. In treating any of these injuries, from headaches to loss of self-esteem, early intervention and a team approach to therapy will give you the best results.

SUGGESTED READINGS

Mandel, S., et al. *Minor Head Trauma.* New York: Springer-Verlag, 1993.

Stoler, D.R., Hill, B.A. *Coping with Mild Brain Injury.* Garden City Park, NY: Avery, 1998.

Wrightson, P., Gronwall, D.M.A. *Mild Head Injury.* New York: Oxford University Press, 1999.

HELPFUL WEB SITES

Post Concussion Syndrome Info & Support Pages
http://www.municipality.co.uk\pcs

***Post Concussion*—The Movie**
http://www.bluewaterfilms.com
An inspirational motion picture written, directed, and edited by David Yoon. Visit the Web site to learn about the film and upcoming screenings.

10

Proof of Alternative Therapies

ANDREW NEWBERG, M.D.

Several years ago, one of my colleagues who practiced acupuncture in his daily clinical activities asked about the possibility of studying how acupuncture works. The reason he came to me is that I had been working on a project to study the effects of meditation on the human brain and therefore had some background in investigating the physiological basis of alternative therapies. The idea of studying acupuncture was a challenging but intriguing proposition. Studying alternative therapies in general is very difficult because of how medical science is usually performed. For example, most traditional therapies for patients with pain have gone the route of empirical testing as guided by the usual principles of the medical profession. This includes developing hypotheses based on current information, testing those hypotheses through a variety of experiments comparing the new therapy with a placebo control group or other existing therapies, and expanding the results to a variety of different disorders and patient populations.

If a physician wants to develop a new drug to help prevent arthritis pain, he or she will explore the effects of current pain-relieving medications, such as aspirin or Ibuprofen, and will work toward developing a drug that acts in a similar manner but possibly has a more direct effect or fewer side effects. After developing the medication, the researcher tests whether it works in human beings by conducting a randomized controlled study. This is the traditional way in which physicians determine if a drug actually works. They randomly assign two groups of patients to receive either the active pill (the new medication) or a pill that looks exactly like the active one but has nothing in it (the placebo). In the ideal study, the patients and physicians are unaware of who is in each of the treatment groups. This is called "blinding" and is very important because studies have shown that when people think that they are being treated for something, they tend to get more of an effect. It is also important that the researchers do not know who is receiving the medications because they may look for more of an effect in patients they know to be receiving the new drug. By comparing the results in a small number of subjects, the researchers can determine if the drug has the desired effect. If it does, they can use the drug on a larger, and sometimes more specific, group of patients. In this case, the researchers may see if the drug works just as well for people with arthritis of the knees as it does for people with arthritis of the hands. Researchers also keep a close eye on the specific measures that are affected by the drugs. Some measures are more subjective: for example, how the person feels, and whether the person feels that he or she has more energy or can do more activities. Other measures are more objective: for example, how much a person can move his or her leg, how much weight he or she can lift, or how much the person can flex his or her back. The difficult part in the development of any therapy is how best to study the therapy, how to measure the therapy, and how to apply the therapy.

With the increasing use of alternative therapies for all kinds of disorders and even for maintaining health, the medical community has realized the importance of studying these therapies in the same rigorous and accurate way as traditional therapies in order to ensure that these therapies are both safe and effective. This has already begun with a growing number of studies reported in the medical journals. In addition to traditional journals, many new alternative therapy journals also have been initiated, including the *Journal of Alternative and Complementary Medicine, Alternative Therapies in Health and Medicine,* and *Complementary Therapies in Medicine.*

The main problem with many alternative therapies is that they present significant challenges to the traditional scientific approaches of study. The biggest problem is that many alternative therapies are based on systems of medicine that do not readily mesh with current Western medical knowledge. For example, when my colleague asked about acupuncture, his first question to me was, "How does it work?" After several hours of explaining that it is based on the body's energy and meridians and special points on the body that affected this flow of energy, I realized that making acupuncture fit into the traditional medical paradigm was almost impossible. We realized, though, that by using some high-tech brain-imaging techniques, we might begin to relate these two systems and help advance both perspectives of the human body.

Other issues that we must face whenever we consider using science to study anything, and alternative therapies in particular, include how we define what the therapy is and how it is supposed to work, who should get the therapy, how we should measure its mechanism and effects, and how someone can use the therapy effectively. This chapter will review these issues and help to show the complexity and need for research in alternative therapies. The most important issue is for researchers to be open to the different paradigms that alternative therapies function within in order to find the most accurate and appropriate ways of studying them.

DEFINING "ALTERNATIVE THERAPY"

The first question that needs to be answered prior to studying alternative therapies is, "Just what exactly is an alternative therapy?" In some broad sense, every therapy that is not currently used is an alternative therapy until it has become part of mainstream medicine. Many therapies that we consider to be mainstream today, especially those such as nutrition, physical therapy, certain types of surgery, certain types of psychotherapy, and even certain medicines, were at one time considered to be alternatives. In fact, it usually required a number of well-constructed scientific studies in order to prove that these approaches actually worked. Only after substantial scrutiny does any kind of therapy become incorporated into the medical practices of most health-care providers. So how do we define what exactly is an alternative therapy? Table 10.1 on page 170 shows a partial list of all the alternative therapies that are commonly used by various practitioners and individuals. Some of these therapies are based on thousands of years of experience, but some only on very limited experience. Some have withstood the rigors of science, and some have failed miserably.

For alternative therapies to become more widely accepted, they will have to be more carefully defined and more thoroughly studied. You might wonder why defining a therapy is so important. Let us take chiropractic approaches to the management of low back pain. From my own personal experience as someone with low back pain, I can list a number of therapeutic interventions that chiropractors perform on patients with low back pain. These include spinal manipulation, spinal adjustments, massage, electrical stimulation, and the use of several machines that stretch and loosen the back. The question now is how to define chiropractic therapy. Is it all of these interventions put together or can some of these interventions be studied separately? And what about the patient/health-care provider relationship? Several studies have shown that this is enhanced in those administering alternative therapies. If we are going to bring science to bear on these approaches, we need to be able to clearly define the interventions, the additional aspects not typically considered part of the therapy, and ultimately the active ingredients of the therapy.

RESEARCH TARGETS

Once we have defined exactly what the alternative therapy is that we're interested in studying, we need to consider the target for that therapy. Some alternative therapies are believed to relieve a number of different problems. Some investigators have begun by exploring therapies that already are at least consistent with the current Western medicine paradigm. For example, herbal therapies are not unlike medicinal therapies in that they are both administered using specified substances and doses. Both herbal preparations and traditional medicines can have side effects and can be used in excess. Because of the similarity, designing studies to investigate the effects of herbal remedies is fairly straightforward and fits into the randomized double-blind study approach. The most important aspect of the similarity is that it is fairly easy to design a placebo control. Usually, it is not difficult to construct a pill that looks exactly like the herbal remedy. But just imagine the difficulty in designing a placebo for something like massage therapy or t'ai chi. How do you do something that looks like the therapy but should not have any effect on the person? Will the control massage therapy consist of simply putting the hands on the patient, massaging the wrong areas, or giving of them a placebo pill that they are told is supposed to be as effective as the massage? Obviously, this is not an easy issue. While the answers to these questions are not immediately forthcoming, with persistence and ingenuity, researchers will hopefully be able to evaluate all types of alternative therapies so that we can eventually know what does and what does not work.

While therapies that fit more easily into the perspective of traditional medicine may be the best "first shot," they may not be the most effective or successful. A certain herbal preparation may help to relieve arthritis pain, but acupuncture may have a more powerful effect. If doctors are more willing to accept the mechanism of the herbal remedy because it is similar to other analgesics, they will more likely give that to patients rather than suggest acupuncture, which is something they may not be able to understand.

Therapeutic touch, for example, is something that is based on the notion of altering certain energies of the body. An article about therapeutic touch was published in the esteemed *Journal of the American Medical Association* (JAMA) about two years ago. There was tremendous controversy over this paper, which essentially found no evidence that practitioners of therapeutic touch actually could detect these energies. For one, the paper had a high school student as the principal author, which was seen by those in the alternative health field as a slap in the face since the medical community seemed to be saying that even a high school student can show that such techniques do not work. However, there were many methodological flaws in the study that arose out of the incompatibility of therapeutic touch with current medical concepts. Whether or not therapeutic touch actually works still awaits further study. The point here is that when studies of alternative therapies show that they work or don't work, it is frequently difficult to determine if the study did in fact measure and show what it intended to show.

Another aspect of alternative therapies is also an important reason that people turn to them. Interestingly, alternative medicine practitioners are frequently perceived to be more caring, more thorough, and more connected to their patients than traditional doctors are to theirs. Alternative medicine practitioners frequently spend more time with patients and give more thorough instructions. This has an important effect on how people perceive the success of those therapies. This is why studies need to be blinded so that practitioners do not know who is getting the actual therapy and who is getting the placebo, because when people receive more attention and more care, they do better regardless of what therapy is used. So it may be difficult to distinguish how well alternative therapies work from how well the practitioners practice. Either way, though, this could have a beneficial effect, if only because the patient feels that he or she is getting better care.

In fairness to JAMA, as well as to the rest of the medical community, there have been an increasing number of studies exploring alternative therapies. Now that alternative therapies have become so universally used by patients, the medical community has begun in earnest to explore exactly how these interventions work and who are the best people to use them on. For example, acupuncture may best be known for its ability to relieve pain; however, it has also been used for a number of other ailments over the past several thousand years in China. So when my colleague asked about studying acupuncture, we had to decide exactly how we would use the acupuncture. Would we study its effects on pain, or would we explore some of its other uses? We decided to focus our research on pain management because it would be easy to measure, both subjectively and objectively.

However, even the measurement of pain is difficult to study from a traditional perspective because pain is so subjectively felt and also can be very different from patient to patient. Pain also can be extremely variable so that the pain level in the morning is significantly different from the pain level in the afternoon. Pain can also be in one spot or spread over a large area. People's tolerance for pain is also very variable so that some people may be in relatively minor pain and feel significant discomfort, whereas others might be in excruciating pain but still be able to live a relatively normal existence.

Researchers have developed a number of ways to measure pain, which ultimately rely on the subjective nature of the experience. And while some of these methods have been very successful, it is still very difficult to compare one person's "seven out of ten" pain with another's. As an example of this difficulty, in my own personal experience, particularly with cardiac patients, I have witnessed some people having what they define as "10/10" chest pain still able to talk fairly normally and even joke with the doctors. We typically define 10/10 pain as being the worst pain imaginable. Other patients may scream and pass out during the insertion of a small needle.

THE IMPORTANCE OF GOOD MEASUREMENT

We ran into the problem of measurement in developing our acupuncture studies. We wanted some objective measure of pain to be able to evaluate when the acupuncture had its greatest effect. While this was effective for assessing pain within an individual subject, we were unable to adequately compare the levels of the subjects' pain with one another. Another problem with pain, especially low back pain, is that it can have several different causes that all feel slightly different. For example, a person may have a disc problem and degenerative changes, both of which can result in discomfort. Treating one aspect of the patient's problem or even trying to evaluate just one aspect may be difficult.

Measurement is not a problem that is exclusive to alternative therapies but is common in all forms of research. The main questions that always have to be answered are "How do I measure what I want to study?" and "Am I measuring what I think that I'm measuring?" These questions are related but are also slightly different. For example, in our study of the effects of meditation, we wanted to measure changes in the brain associated with the feeling of oneness experienced by the practitioner. In order to do this, we decided to use a high-tech imaging camera called SPECT (single photon emission computed tomography). This instrument, which we also used in our acupuncture study, can be used to measure blood flow in the brain. It turns out that the brain delivers more blood to an active area than an inactive area. So blood flow is associated with the level of activity. But we have to do more than just measure the blood flow during meditation, we have to compare it with some "resting" state or other state of the brain in order to see the difference. So we had people remain in a normal waking state for the baseline scan and then had them meditate for the second scan. In this way, we measured how the blood flow in the brain changed during meditation and concluded that these were the changes associated with meditation. We had measured changes based on what we were interested in studying. However, other questions remained: Did we, in fact, measure the meditative state? How do we know that the person isn't sleeping? How do we know that we captured the highest level of the person's meditation? What about changes in blood flow? We were very interested in certain brain structures that might actually be inhibited or shut down by other structures. If there is an increase in inhibition, would that turn up as increased or decreased blood flow?

Fortunately, many of these issues are already well known and described in the brain-imaging literature. Thus, we felt very comfortable stating that certain areas of the brain were activated and certain areas deactived during meditation. We also felt comfortable that we had measured the meditative state, since we had worked out a specific observable signal that the meditator would do that would inform us when to take the meditation scan. Since the subjects would have to be awake in order to perform this signal, we knew that they had to be awake. Future studies might try to compare the brain scans with other measures to determine the level and extent of the meditation. We might measure changes in electrical activity in the brain, something that we know is distinct during meditation. If we are ultimately interested in how meditation affects our bodies, we may have to add measures of heart rate, blood pressure, and hormone and immune functions. So measuring things in general is not always straightforward.

Another example of measurement difficulties can be found in the acupuncture studies we performed using SPECT imaging. Each of the patients we studied had suffered from a chronic pain condition for at least two years. These patients did not respond to traditional medical therapy, including nonsteroidal anti-inflammatory medications, narcotics, or tricyclic analgesics. Nor did they respond to physical therapy or steroid injections. However, each of the patients responded very well to acupuncture treatment. When the patients first arrived at our laboratory, we obtained a subjective assessment of pain using a ten-digit score test. The first assessment was the pre-acupuncture level of pain. The patients each underwent an acupuncture technique with the points selected that had been previously used in past treatments of the patient. They had another assessment when they perceived significant relief from the pain (the post-acupuncture level of pain). The patients had a SPECT scan at the time they were experiencing their typical pain and then a second one after relief of their pain. While their pain levels were significantly improved (patients went from an average of 7.6 to 3 out of 10) after the acupuncture, it was the scans that were particularly important. If we could demonstrate a change, then we would be able to show that acupuncture does do something—something that affects us on a very basic level within the brain itself. The most striking change we observed in every patient was in a part of the brain called the thalamus (there are actually two thalami, one on the left and one on the right). (See Figure 10.1.) This structure has been shown to be intimately involved in the perception of pain. When the patients were experiencing pain, their thalami showed a strong asymmetry (one side was more active than the other). However, after acupuncture, the asymmetry either went away or sometimes actually went in the other direction.

Clearly something was happening, but we wondered what these changes actually measured. Did these changes reflect the effects of acupuncture that resulted in a relief of pain, or did we measure the relief of pain directly and the acupuncture actually worked by some other mechanism? Part of the problem with evaluating alternative therapies is that their mechanisms are not clearly established in many circumstances. We can measure the clinical effects such as whether certain herbal ther-

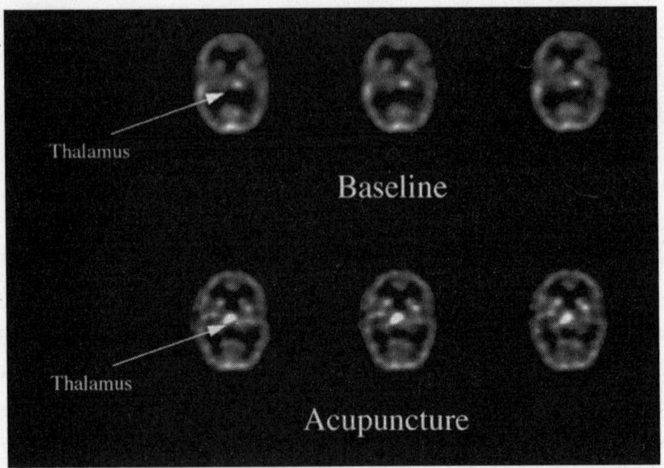

FIGURE 10.1
Brain Scan images of a subject with pain (baseline) and then with relief of pain after treatment with acupuncture. The more white present in the area of the brain, the more active the area is, or the less pain.

apies help cure cold symptoms. However, we might also try to measure physiological changes that might show how the intervention works biologically such as by improving the function of immune cells.

Some diseases are also easier to study. After all, an intervention designed to lower blood pressure should be easy to evaluate. We simply have to measure the blood pressure before and after therapy. But even that may not be so simple. Studies have shown that when people first arrive at a doctor's office, their blood pressure goes up. So if we measure the blood pressure initially, have someone meditate or undergo acupuncture, and then measure the blood pressure again, how do we know if the blood pressure improvement is related to the person getting used to being with the doctor and not related to the therapy? Of course there are ways around these problems, but researchers studying alternative therapies need to be aware of the many problems that arise from doing research.

The other important measurement issue is what constitutes the appropriate control group. We have already touched on this issue above, but it is so crucial to good research that it is necessary to explore it in relation to measurement. After all, making a good measurement is tantamount to showing if something works. A fascinating example of this is in acupuncture therapy for pain. Acupuncture in the right place has been shown to be effective in relieving pain in approximately 60 to 70 percent of patients. Compared with a placebo pill, acupuncture would be a significant improvement, since placebo has been shown to work in approximately 20 percent of cases. But some investigators have suggested that the appropriate comparison is "sham acupuncture" or acupuncture in the wrong place. This ensures that the subject does not experience a benefit simply from contact with the physician or because he or she thinks that the acupuncture will work. The problem is that sham acupuncture has approximately a 40- to 50-percent rate of effectiveness. Trying to demonstrate a beneficial effect of acupuncture in comparison to sham acupuncture will obviously be much more difficult and require a much larger number of cases.

The question then is, what should be the best control? The control group should have all the components of the intervention without actually doing anything. There continues to be debate in the acupuncture world about the best way to approach these studies. This issue of the appropriate comparison groups will be a critical one to grapple with for researchers attempting to determine the efficacy and mechanism of alternative therapies.

STUDYING THE EFFECTIVENESS OF ALTERNATIVE THERAPIES

Clinical studies will be crucial in determining which alternative therapies are the most beneficial for which diseases. In traditional medical studies, usually a limited group of patients is selected. For example, if a study of how a drug improves pain is undertaken, the investigators usually select one type of pain syndrome such as surgical pain, arthritis pain, or nerve pain. Researchers typically have to determine the best population of patients to study and try to eliminate other confounding issues. For example, if some of the pain patients have depression or anxiety problems, this might complicate the ability to determine whether the drug the researchers are studying is effective. Furthermore, some types of pain, such as surgical pain, may go away without treatment, some types of pain may get progressively worse over time, and some types of pain may come and go. Each of these characteristics of pain must be taken into account.

The most appropriate clinical problems must be studied first and must be based on current knowledge. If a certain herbal therapy has demonstrated some benefit in treating depression, then a large scale study of depressed patients would be a good first step. Future studies might identify patients with relapsing depression or determine if the herbal therapy helps prevent relapse. Studies might also explore how this herbal therapy affects patients with related psychological problems, such as anxiety, or try to determine if the herbal therapy prevents depression in patients with chronic illness. With these issues in mind, it would not make sense to use the herbal preparation in the treatment of diabetes as an initial target for study.

Dose determination is a crucial issue in any therapy and especially in alternative therapies. Too much or too little of any therapy may not yield a beneficial effect and may increase the risk of side effects or the risk of worsening a condition not adequately treated. Another problem with alternative therapies is that they typically do not have standardized doses. In the study of a blood pressure drug, investigators can study a scale of doses and determine where the best effects exist and may find that the dose can be increased depending on the situation. People who have mildly increased blood pressure may get a low dose compared with people who have very high blood pressure. But since many alternative therapies have multiple components and varying amounts of those components, it is more difficult to determine the best dose. In herbal preparations, there is sometimes a wide variability in the amount of the active ingredients. In acupuncture treatments, there may be differences in how many points are used and how often the therapy is administered.

Selecting the appropriate measures and outcomes is also important. A therapy may decrease the level of pain but not the level of disability. Also, the time of follow-up is important since some therapies may work in the short term but lose their benefits over a longer period of time.

Adverse reactions are always a critical issue in medical research and are similarly important in the study of alternative therapies. Ideally, herbal preparations should be treated as drugs with both active ingredients and side effects. Some of the side effects might be particularly problematic. The safety of such therapies must also be explored in pregnancy and in children. Long-term risks such as cancer should also be considered, especially with herbal preparations that contain hormone-related ingredients.

It will be the clinical trials that ultimately establish or reject the use of various alternative therapies in medical practice. For this reason, well-performed clinical trials will be critical to the future use of alternative therapies and for their incorporation into the mainstream practice of the health-care field.

HOW DO ALTERNATIVE THERAPIES WORK?

This aspect of the study of alternative therapies will have important implications for their use in medical practice and for developing future therapies. By establishing how various alternative therapies actually work and where they work in the body, we will enhance our knowledge of these therapies as well as our knowledge of the human body. Studies that search for mechanisms will usually have to relate the therapies to the more traditional understanding of the human body and human diseases. Understanding acupuncture in the treatment of pain will require the

TABLE 10.1 RESEARCH SUMMARIES OF SOME COMPLEMENTARY AND ALTERNATIVE THERAPIES

Therapy	Current State of Research
Acupuncture	Most effective for pain management; overall mechanism also studied, but not yet clear.
Aromatherapy	Demonstrated to be effective for certain problems, such as pain, anxiety, and wound healing.
Ayurveda	Extensive tradition with many practices having significant benefit while others are not well tested.
Biofeedback	Successful for a number of physical and psychological disorders.
Chiropractic	Benefits certain types of specific disorders, such as low back pain.
Folk Remedies	Varying degrees of evidence to suggest that what people have traditionally done has some benefit.
Healing Touch	Appears to have some benefits, although the mechanism of action is controversial.
Herbal Medicine	Some herbs are well tested; however, many preparations are untested and have potential side effects and drug interactions.
Homeopathy	Several studies have demonstrated effectiveness, but underlying principles are not well tested.
Imagery	Beneficial for relaxation and possibly for disorders such as depression and anxiety.
Light Therapy	May have benefits for seasonal affective disorder (SAD).
Massage	Beneficial for relaxation and related effects.
Meditation	Induces relaxation, lowers heart rate, and lowers blood pressure.
Naturopathic	Represents an overall approach to health based on a number of traditional and alternative principles.
Osteopathy	Extensive practice with a number of beneficial effects from both the traditional and alternative components.
Prayer	Beneficial for coping, psychological state, and some physical health problems; intercessory prayer of uncertain value.
Qigong (Chi Kung)	Beneficial for cardiovascular disease, aging, cancer, and diabetes, but mechanism is not based in traditional medicine.
Vitamins	Some vitamins prevent disease, and everyone needs enough; some high-dose regimens are less well tested.
Yoga	Good for stress management and has demonstrated other health benefits.

evaluation of the brain mechanisms and pain pathways in the body before, during, and after acupuncture therapy. Measures of nerve activity and brain function will help to establish whether or not these therapies have a physiological effect that can be linked to the clinical effects.

Our laboratory, as well as others, has explored the mechanisms of various interventions such as acupuncture and meditation. These studies have helped to link these therapies to the specific parts of the body and brain that help to alter different disease processes. The field of psychoneuroimmunology and related fields help to link together what happens in the brain and the body.

As the clinical studies demonstrate specific benefits and/or adverse effects of alternative therapies, science can specifically explore the mechanisms underlying these effects. This will be of prime importance for establishing the efficacy of alternative therapies. As much as clinical responses can demonstrate the usefulness of alternative therapies, seeing how they work provides a crucial piece of the puzzle to determine when and how such therapies can be used.

THE FUTURE OF ALTERNATIVE THERAPIES

The future is very bright for the scientific study of alternative therapies. However, researchers will require attention to detail and a significant effort to ensure that good science is performed while preserving the essential components of the alternative therapy. Because of the tremendous public interest in alternative therapies, many top scientists have directed their attention toward finding out which therapies are the best and how they work. There has also been the development of a center for alternative medicine at the National Institutes of Health. The creation of this center, and the expansion of good researchers in this field, will hopefully ensure that alternative therapies play a prominent role in the future of medical research.

SUGGESTED READINGS

Fontanarosa, Phil B. *Alternative Medicine: An Objective Assessment.* Chicago: American Medical Association, 2000.

Koenig, Harold G. *Handbook on Religion and Health.* New York: Oxford University Press, 2001.

Micozzi, Marc S. *Fundamentals of Complementary and Alternative Medicine.* New York: Churchill Livingston, 1996.

HELPFUL WEB SITES

Center for Mind-Body Medicine
http://www.cmbm.org/

HerbMed
http://www.herbmed.org/

National Center for Complementary and Alternative Medicines/ National Institutes of Health
http://nccam.nih.gov/

Research Council for Complementary Medicine
http://www.rccm.org.uk/cisc.htm

University of Pennsylvania
http://www.uphs.upenn.edu/progdev/compmed/index.html

11

Acupuncture and Trigger-Point Therapy

When a Needle Is Not a Needle

JENNIFER CHU, M.D.

Patient Profile

At age forty-eight, Yolanda had a normal life, working full-time and possessing full capacity to participate in recreational and social activities. Then, a snowboarding accident left her with pain in her neck and right shoulder and radiating pain down both arms. The discomfort caused by the accident was exacerbated by Yolanda's protective posture, which kept the injured muscles relatively immobilized but resulted in stiffening with significant limitations in movement. Physical therapy was not successful, and a manipulation under anesthesia followed by four months of physiotherapy was required to restore mobility in her right shoulder. During this time, the pain produced considerable disabilities in Yolanda's family and home responsibilities, recreational activities, social and occupational activities, as well as life-support activities such as sleeping.

Over the course of four years, Yolanda sought pain relief from nine medical practitioners, including two orthopedists, one rheumatologist, one spinal and cranial neurosurgeon, one neurologist, one physiatrist/acupuncturist, two physical therapists, and one chiropractor. Medications and other forms of therapy prescribed included Flexeril, Elavil, Ultram, trigger-point injections, and exercise, including swimming and yoga. Despite undergoing many forms of standard treatments, Yolanda remained in significant pain.

Having exhausted "conventional" treatments, she began researching other options on the Internet. It was through a connection made this way that she set up an appointment with the author, who subsequently evaluated her at the Hospital of the University of Pennsylvania. An MRI revealed bulging discs at the C3-C4, C5-C6, and C6-C7 levels at the neck spine. The most involved nerve roots on electromyography (EMG) were also the C4, C5, C6, and C7 nerve roots. The multiple spinal nerve root injuries were related to a traction/transient compression/distortion type injury of these nerve roots against underlying bones or bulging discs of the cervical spine.

Since Yolanda's symptoms were those of nerve-related muscle pain, she was an ideal candidate to receive treatments pioneered by the author, known as automated twitch-obtaining intramuscular stimulation (ATOIMS) and electrical twitch-obtaining intramuscular stimulation (ETOIMS) treatments. She achieved remarkable pain relief after two sessions and then continued treatments on a biweekly basis. During treatment, which involves the stimulation of muscles with a needle at specific points to produce a contraction or twitch, the muscles noted to be most difficult to "twitch" were those that were damaged in her accident. This was due to chronic tightness of the muscles resulting from chronic nerve root irritation. By the tenth treatment, Yolanda had improved significantly. She was able to wean the treatments to once a month and has remained in therapy for over two years. Her quality of life has improved substantially. She is able to continue working full-time and to enjoy social and recreational activities once again.

~

NERVE-RELATED muscle injuries like those suffered by Yolanda are all too common, for young and old alike. Muscles surrounding injured nerves go into spasm to protect the nerves, which serves to further irritate the nerves and continues a cycle of increasing pain and muscle tightening.

There are a number of methods of treatment currently available to alleviate the discomfort caused by musculoskeletal pain.

THE THEORY OF ACUPUNCTURE

Acupuncture is one of the less mainstream pain-relieving methods. Awareness of this therapy began in the United States in the early 1970s and has become more popular with the rising interest in alternative medicine. It has been widely used in China and elsewhere for thousands of years. The earliest Chinese medical classic, *Huangdi Nei Jing,* was compiled between 500 and 300 B.C. This text summarizes the medical experience and theoretical knowledge of the ancient Chinese and describes acupuncture points and needling methods.

Acupuncture is used in traditional Chinese medicine to prevent and treat disease by puncturing certain points on the body with needles. The theory behind traditional acupuncture is that excessive energy systems in some body areas and deficient energy systems in complementary areas are balanced to restore the body to its original healthy state. The energy-balancing concept of yin/yang holds that every object in the universe consists of two opposite aspects that are in conflict but are interdependent. Characteristics such as quiescence, coldness, downward direction, inward position, dimness, lack of strength, inhibition, and slowness pertain to yin. Anything that is moving, hot, in an upward direction, exterior position, bright, excited, rapid, unsubstantial, and so on, belongs to yang. The tissues and organs of the human body may pertain either to yin or yang, according to their relative locations and functions. Viewing the body as a whole, the trunk surface and the four extremities being on the exterior pertain to yang. The organs are inside the body and are therefore yin. The two aspects of yin and yang are not fixed but are in a state of constant motion. For instance, depletion of yin leads to excess of yang, while deficiency of yang results in too much yin. Under normal conditions, these opposites maintain a relative balance. Under abnormal conditions, discomfort or disease results because of inequality of yin and yang.

Since the occurrence of a disease is the outcome of imbalance between yin and yang, all the methods of treatment should aim at reconciling the two and restoring them to a condition of relative balance. This is accomplished through manual insertion of a wiry acupuncture needle at designated acupuncture points on energy channels, or "meridians," along which energy flows within the body. There are 14 such meridians, and the 365 acupuncture points lie along these meridians. (See figures

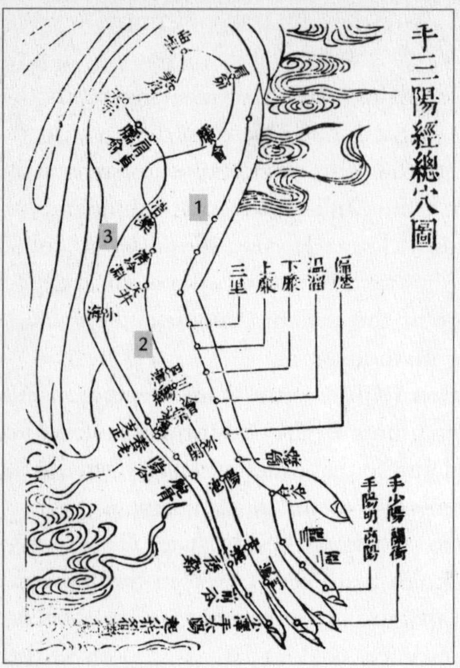

FIGURE 11.1
Segments of some of the acupuncture meridians along the upper limb: 1) large-intestine meridian (in the line of the index finger) for treating disorders along this channel including those of the large intestine, lungs, and skin; 2) triple-burner meridian (along the back of the upper limb) for disorders of the thoracic, abdominal, and pelvic organs; 3) small-intestine meridian (in the line of the little finger) for treatment of musculoskeletal pain along this meridian.

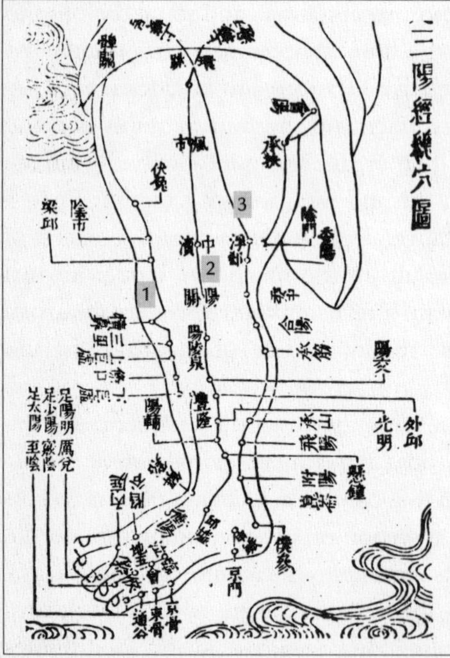

FIGURE 11.2
Segments of some of the acupuncture meridians along the lower limb: 1) stomach meridian (in the middle of the front of the limb) for treating head, neck, and gastrointestinal and pelvic disorders; 2) gallbladder meridian runs along the outer aspect of the limb (in the line of the fourth digit) and is used for liver and gallbladder disorders and musculoskeletal pain; 3) bladder meridian (in the line of the little toe and along the middle of the back of the limb) for treatment of kidney, urogenital, and musculoskeletal disorders along this region.

11.1 and 11.2) The meridians traverse the limbs, trunk, and face. In an acupuncture treatment, points on the right side may be selected to treat disorders of the left side and vice versa, while points on the lower portion of the body may be selected to treat disorders of the upper portion and vice versa. All of these methods are based on the concept of regarding the body as an organic whole. The aim of treatment is to readjust the relationship of yin and yang and to promote circulation of *qi* (energy) and blood.

Many disorders are claimed to be treatable by acupuncture; the most common use of acupuncture is in the treatment of muscloskeletal pain. The scientific basis for acupuncture in pain treatment is based on needle activation of the sensory receptors or small nerve fibers of A delta and C in size. Nerve fibers are classified by size according to whether they originate in skin or muscle; myelin, which is the blanket surrounding the nerve, allows the nerve to conduct faster. Large myelinated A beta (skin) or type I (muscle) carry touch and deep sensations, respectively. Small myelinated A delta (skin) or types II and III (muscle) carry pain; the smallest myelinated C (skin) and type IV (muscle) carry pain. Types II, III, IV, and C also carry non-painful messages. On needle stimulation of skin or muscle, an impulse is sent to the spinal cord via type II and type III afferent nerves (these small myelinated afferent nerves carry sensory information toward the spinal cord). Type II afferent nerves signal the needling sensations of numbness called *De Qi,* and type III afferent nerves convey the feeling of fullness (having a sensation). Soreness is also felt that is carried by unmyelinated type IV afferent nerves from the muscle (but soreness usually is not part of the *De Qi* sensations). In acupuncture points where there are no muscles (for example, in a fingertip), different nerve fibers may be stimulated. The nerves then relay information in the spinal cord to the pain-conducting anterolateral tract, which projects to one of the three centers—the spinal cord, the mid-brain, or the hypothalamus-pituitary complex in the upper part of the brain.

The practical significance of this three-level system is as follows: When needles are placed close to the site of the pain, or in the tender (trigger or bone) points, they are maximizing the segmental circuits in the spinal cord while also bringing in cells from the other two centers. When needles are placed in distal points far away from the painful region, they activate the mid-brain and hypothalams-pituitary cells without the benefit of local segmental effects. Local segmental needling usually gives a more intensive analgesic effect than distal non-segmental needling because it uses all three centers. Generally, the two kinds of needling (local and distal) are used together to enhance each other. Low-frequency high-intensity needling works through the endorphin system and acts in all three centers, while a high-frequency with low-intensity needling activates only the spinal cord, bypassing the endorphin system. Low frequency has been claimed to produce an analgesic effect of slower onset and, more important, of long duration, outlasting the twenty-minute stimulation session by thirty minutes to many hours. Also, the effects are cumulative, becoming increasingly better after several treatments. The high-frequency stimulation–induced analgesic effect, in contrast, is rapid in onset, very short-lasting, and has no cumulative effects.

To block incoming painful information, the spinal cord center uses *enkephalin* and *dynorphin*. The mid-brain center uses enkephalin to activate the system that is responsible for inhibition of spinal cord pain transmission using other naturally occuring chemicals such as serotonin and epinephrine. The third center, the hypothalamus-pituitary area, releases beta endorphin into the blood and cerebral spinal fluid to cause analgesia at a distance. Thus, all three endorphins (enkephalin, beta endorphin, and dynorphin) as well as serotonin and epinephrine have a role in acupuncture's analgesic effects.

Prevailing wisdom holds that the release of endorphins from these three centers (spinal cord, mid-brain, and hypothalamus-pituary) is what actually affords relief from pain with acupuncture methods. However, endorphin release can also be found with painful stimuli, vigorous exercise, and relaxation training, and is therefore not specific to acupuncture. As it is insertion of a needle that is specific to acupuncture, the resulting local effects of that needle insertion into muscle are important to understand.

As pain relief can be achieved through acupuncture, it is worth examining the physiological benefits of this kind of therapy. Musculoskeletal pain is primarily due to shortening of the muscle fibers from nerve root irritation making the muscles hard and even swollen, and it is commonly known to be helped by physical methods that mobilize muscle tissue such as massage, exercise, or stretching. Therefore, in using a needle to achieve pain relief, acupuncture effects may depend on the local stimulating effects of the needle on penetrating the muscle.

ELICITING MUSCLE TWITCHES

Traditional acupuncture describes a subjective sensation of numbness, pressure, heaviness, soreness, or distention resulting from needle placement at tender acupuncture points. However, similar sensations are also described in the identification of muscle trigger points and in needling muscle tissue at tender points during electromyography (EMG), a diagnostic test for nerve and muscle disorders. It consists of recording muscle wave forms using a monopolar needle electrode inserted into the muscle.

The tender points in a muscle have been shown by EMG to be "motor end-plate zones" (MEPZs) or nerve-muscle junction points, where a nerve tells its muscle what to do. On needling the MEPZs, muscle twitches can be elicited. The twitch is a sudden, abrupt contraction of parts of the muscle or the whole muscle. Very minute twitches are easily recordable with the EMG needle, whereas large twitches are easily felt or are grossly visible. The MEPZs that most readily produce twitches are usually found along the depressed edges of taut bands, ropes, or nodes within the muscle and along linear grooves within or between the muscles. Commonly, traditional acupuncture points also are located in similar locations within the muscle. Acupuncture points, trigger points, and MEPZs are identical points that, if needled, provide similar pain relief. Therefore, to treat muscle pain, it stands to reason to treat where the muscle is tender and not where the traditional acupuncture points are present as on the meridians.

Difference in the clinical effects upon needling these points depends on the type of needle used and the ease with which forceful muscle twitches can be elicited with such a needle. The firmer and stronger monopolar EMG electrode is more useful than the wiry acupuncture needle in eliciting muscle twitches. The monopolar EMG electrode can penetrate deep into tissues to stimulate MEPZs within the depths of the muscle, and this one single needle can withstand repeated use in stimulating multiple points in multiple areas during a treatment session. Twitch elicitation is essential to exercise and mobilize muscle tissues, especially the deep muscle fibers.

Traditional acupuncture is not the most suitable method to achieve this type of result because clinically noticeable muscle twitches that are grossly visible with enough force to shake or move the joint do not typically occur. These types of twitches occur on needling the muscle where there may be intramuscular bands/knots in the muscle, especially when accompanied by tenderness at such a point. Also, lack of tensile strength of the thin and wiry acupuncture needle is not useful for consistently eliciting twitches with slow manual insertion of the needle. Twitches can occur by using this needle with a technique termed intramuscular stimulation (IMS). As described by Dr. Chan Gunn, IMS uses a plunger to manually force the acupuncture needle into a muscle at tender points within the muscle, and oscillatory (back-and-forth movements) methods are also used to provide a series of stimuli. However, even with this method, the acupuncture needle is not ideal for oscillation purposes because with repeated oscillations, the acupuncture needle's original trajectory deflects away from the targeted MEPZs, especially when the muscle tightens up. Also, mechanical stimulation of intramuscular terminal nerve fibers from the oscillatory needle movements resulting in twitches moves tissues so that the same tissue is not stimulated with each needle oscillation. Since tissues have a tendency to adhere to the bare stainless-steel shaft of this type of needle during the oscillatory needle movements, the needle will bend, twist, or corkscrew when pushed into stiff and thick skin and muscle tissue.

It is notable, however, that twitch elicitation may occur with EMG performed with a standard monopolar needle electrode at similar points as used in acupuncture. Intramuscular needle movement and needle diameter influence twitch elicitation during EMG. The standard monopolar EMG needle electrode measures 16/1000 inch in diameter and is larger, stronger, and more efficient for skin and muscle penetration than an acupuncture needle, whose diameter is approximately 10/1000 inch. The Teflon coat on the shaft of the monopolar EMG needle allows smooth insertion of the needle into muscle tissue and limits electrical exposure to its tip. There is also easy maneuverability of this needle within the muscle, which facilitates oscillation of the needle, producing twitches.

Another treatment for muscle pain associated with tender trigger points is the injection of local anesthetics such as lidocaine into the corresponding points. The hypodermic needle used for injecting trigger points has sufficient strength to penetrate deep into tissue. Still, its beveled edge, which can be destructive to tissues, limits oscillation within muscles. Additionally, the twitch that is necessary for pain relief is suppressed when local anesthetics are injected, negating the potential benefits of using the needle. Therefore, the therapeutic significance of a twitch remains unrecognized with trigger-point injections. Even the relief afforded by the local anesthetics is short lived, since when the effects of local anesthetics dissipate, the muscle pain returns. This is because the cause of the pain, which is muscle shortening from nerve irritation or nerve damage, still has not been treated. The muscle shortening is responsible for the pain symptoms and can be detected on feeling the affected muscles for the presence of intramuscular bands/knots that will remain hard, swollen, and tender. The range of motion of joints over which the affected muscles cross over also remains limited.

Dr. Gunn's hypothesis is that the degeneration of spinal discs and joints caused by aging produces rough surfaces that irritate the nerve roots. This, in turn, causes muscle fibers to shorten and tighten. The resultant pain is from the traction effect of shortened muscle fibers on nerves and blood vessels within the muscle as well as on the tendons, bones, intervertebral discs, and joints. The traction effect of muscle fibers on nerves leads to more irritation of the nerves, causing more muscle-fiber shortening, which initiates a vicious cycle.

IMS achieved pain relief by causing immediate local muscle-fiber relaxation through oscillation, the twisting and turning motions of the intramuscularly inserted acupuncture needle. However, these pain-relief effects are very limited compared with those associated with a new and improved method of intramuscular stimulation termed twitch-obtaining intramuscular stimulation (TOIMS).

Twitch-Obtaining Intramuscular Stimulation (TOIMS)

As suggested by the name, TOIMS is similar to IMS in that a needle is inserted into muscle fibers. The difference between the two methods lies in the fact that TOIMS seeks to elicit a twitch of the related muscle as evidence of effective muscle contraction and relaxation. This leads to stretching of denervation-induced shortened muscle fibers in the immediate surroundings of those muscle fibers involved in the twitch. TOIMS treatments produce twitches by stimulating the intramuscular nerve terminals, branches, or nerve trunks and/or muscle.

The tight areas can be defined from the presence of tender intramuscular bands/knots, and these areas are where the irritated or degenerating nerves that cause muscles to shorten are present. When such nerves are stimulated, twitch-associated contraction and subsequent relaxation in these regions produce effective focal stretching to the adjacent shortened muscle fibers. The best therapy results are associated with twitch forces large enough to move or shake the joint over which the treated muscle crosses.

The force of the twitch can give an indication about the health status of the nerve and muscle tissue at the treated areas. When the nerve and muscle tissue is not too healthy or if the muscle fibers are too short, it does not respond well to mechanical or electrical stimulation. In such instances, the force of the twitch is small, since only a few muscle fibers will be contracting to result in a twitch. If the muscle is scarred, or fibrotic, there will be no twitches. On the other hand, when the nerve and muscle tissue at the treated areas is healthier, the resulting twitch may visibly shake the joint over which it crosses. Excessively large-force twitches that move the joint in the direction of action of the treated muscle are the most useful twitches for effective therapy. These large-force twitches indicate the presence of supersensitivity to mechanical or electrical stimulation of the nerve tissues at that area. Ability to locate and elicit such twitches is the key to pain reduction, since these twitches can effectively exercise, mobilize, and stretch large areas of tight muscle tissue. Circulation is essential for all tissues to heal well, and the large-force twitches prepare the muscle to receive adequate amounts of blood. This concept is essential for aiding in the regeneration of nerves and muscles.

All of these factors aid in immediate pain relief. Over time, these beneficial effects aid in healing nerve and muscle tissue, decreasing or ending the cycles of pain that normally render the injury permanent. As the irritated nerves heal through nerve regeneration, tenderness in the muscles disappears, the muscles become softer and less swollen, and the range of motion in the affected segments improves. On the other hand, if muscle tissue is so tight that large-force twitches cannot be elicited, the treatments may be painful, and there is no pain relief. The chance of obtaining pain relief with the TOIMS method in such patients is decreased. If no pain relief is achieved after four to five TOIMS treatments, treatments may be discontinued. As long as there is pain relief with objective signs of improvement, treatments can be continued periodically on an indefinite basis. This is because the nerve root irritation due to degeneration of the spine, usually initiated by trauma, is an ongoing process.

When irritation of bilateral multiple spinal nerve roots occurs secondary to acute or cumulative trauma, multiple trigger points can result and treatments cannot be directed only to the nerves. Normally given for this type of diffuse pain, medications often have side effects that can lead to decreased brain and body functions. This type of pain is responsive to IMS but is difficult and inefficient to treat with manual insertion and oscillation of a needle due to the diffuseness of the pain. It is also a labor- and time-intensive treatment for the physician to perform, and the physician can be subjected to repetitive stress injuries. Automation of this process was thus necessary to insert, oscillate, and retract the needle from the muscle.

ATOIMS AND ETOIMS Automated twitch-obtaining intramuscular stimulation (ATOIMS) utilizes a handheld custom device. The device facilitates intensive treatments to multiple points in multiple muscles of patients with diffuse nerve-related chronic muscle pain. Since the ATOIMS device regulates and maintains only one smooth trajectory for the oscillating pin, it minimizes tissue trauma, treatment pain, and post-treatment pain. It also improves reliability, efficiency, and accuracy of treatment. It is essential for treatment of areas with very stiff and tight muscle tissue. Use of the device also decreases the risk of cumulative and repetitive stress injury to the treating physician.

Although this device is very effective, the addition of a small electrical charge, similar to that furnished by the EMG diagnostic machine, seemed a logical next step in the evolution of this twitch-obtaining therapy. Electrical excitation of nerves is more powerful than mechanical stimulation in consistently evoking twitches. The development of electrical twitch-obtaining intramuscular stimulation (ETOIMS) increased both the total number and force of elicited twitches. The author has shown that patients suffering from myofascial pain and fibromyalgia with multiple trigger points get more effective pain relief with ETOIMS, which is attributed to the ease of generating large-force twitches.

The most effective type of stretching of muscle fibers shortened due to nerve injury is that which occurs in the immediate vicinity of the affected muscle fibers. Electrical fields have a steep decay with increased distance from the electrical stimulus source. Thus, ETOIMS and ATOIMS have the capacity to excite only the intramuscular nerve branches closest to the stimulating electrode of the devices. These methods concentrate the stretch effects closer to where muscle fibers are shortened. Therefore, the effects are more specific and therapeutic than surface electrical stimulation used by physical therapists.

Transcutaneous electrical nerve stimulation (TENS) achieves pain relief by stimulating large nerve fibers in the skin that close a "pain gate" in the spinal cord. Closing this gate prevents painful impulses from reaching the brain. As muscle has larger nerve fibers than skin, stimulation of these nerves by ETOIMS-induced twitches has more potential than TENS in closing the pain gate.

The pain-relieving effects of percutaneous electrical nerve stimulation (PENS), or electrical acupuncture, may be similar to ETOIMS. With PENS, electrical stimulation of only very superficial MEPZs occurs, since the acupuncture needle used in PENS cannot deeply penetrate muscle for effective deep stimulation. Also, the stainless-steel shaft of the acupuncture needle conducts electricity and stimulates tissues surrounding the needle shaft. The treatment time with these procedures is arbitrary and is usually in the range of ten to twenty minutes. With ETOIMS, the stimulation is two seconds per point, and the micro-stimulation is focused only on intramuscular nerves close to the tip of the needle, since the entire shaft is coated with Teflon. In theory, this would increase therapeutic effectiveness of ETOIMS while decreasing the potential for tissue damage, compared with electrical stimulation using noncoated stainless-steel needles.

Spinal nerve root degeneration and related muscle fiber shortening from aging can recur or become progressive with further acute or chronic repetitive trauma to the spinal nerve roots, as with Yolanda in the patient profile at the beginning of this chapter. Pain-relieving anti-inflammatories (steroids and nonsteroidal medications), muscle relaxants, and narcotics can help the pain temporarily but do not affect the cause of the muscle pain. That pain may be due to deep muscle tightness at multiple points in muscles throughout the body. Therefore, it is important that treatments for such conditions treat the cause of the problem and also are safe and effective, especially for repetitive long-term use.

SUGGESTED READINGS

Chu, J. "Putting It All Together: Treatment Templates and Case Studies—Electrical Twitch Obtaining Intramuscular Stimulation," in Mayor D (ed), *Electroacupuncture*. London: Harcourt Health Sciences, 2002.

A list of appropriate references of the author's publications is available upon request at www.painfree-international.org

HELPFUL WEB SITE

Painfree International Charitable Foundation
http://www.painfree-international.org
The Web site of the charitable foundation formed by patients of Jennifer Chu, M.D.

12

Bodywork

JANO COHEN

By using bodywork techniques, you can reduce many of the effects of physical trauma. The greater your physical flexibility and mobility, the more likely it is that your pain and fatigue will be less. The techniques described in this chapter can be used to complement the medical care you are receiving. They may help bring relief from your symptoms, and they usually are pleasurable. You may want to sample several disciplines to find the ones that work best for you.

"Bodywork" is a general term that refers to the full range of touch therapies. The bodywork techniques described in this chapter can be grouped into four major categories: touch and manipulation; movement education and reeducation; energetic healing; and awareness training, or mind-body control. All of these approaches offer a number of techniques that may help you heal, decrease your pain, and restore your body to its normal level of activity by improving your flexibility and mobility.

After you are injured, performing your daily tasks of living becomes more difficult. Initially, you may have to rest for long periods, and during this inactivity your body will lose elasticity, tone, and liveliness. Then you may move unconsciously in ways that actually increase your symptoms. For example, if you brace yourself to avoid pain, your movement becomes tense and uncoordinated and may put extra pressure on certain parts of your body. Or you may exert too much force to move your body, which increases your pain. You may get very tired and slump; this tightens muscles in the front of your spine and lets the ones in the back go slack. This imbalance distorts the spine and results in extra pressure on discs and nerves. Victims of whiplash often repeatedly stiffen their necks during activity long after the initial injury; others may favor a sprained ankle long after it has healed.

Studying bodywork techniques can help you become aware of your destructive movement habits and give you a process to change these habits. You can learn better ways to lift things, do your work, exercise, and move without increasing your pain. You can reduce the effort you use to move, which will help conserve your energy. You can learn not to lock parts of your body together or push them to the end of their range of movement. You can move your whole body in a more coordinated way. You also can learn to rest in more constructive ways and bring new awareness to your body to help it heal.

Always check with your doctors as well as your bodywork teacher or practitioner to see if a technique is safe for you. Some health conditions could cause certain movements or therapeutic techniques to slow your healing or harm your health. These conditions may include bruises, open wounds, infection, excessive edema, advanced diabetes, metastatic cancer, heart disease, or bleeding disorders. If you have a history of physical violence or abuse, consult a mental-health practitioner before trying any form of treatment that might make you uncomfortable or stimulate unpleasant memories.

TOUCH AND MANIPULATION

Many forms of touch therapy, or manual therapy, are available. The touch therapies described in this chapter include osteopathic manipulation, massage, and techniques that promote mobility of the connective tissue. Chiropractic care and acupuncture are described in other chapters.

GOALS OF BODYWORK	
To Improve Your	**To Reduce Your**
breathing	anxiety and stress
circulation	blood pressure and toxicity
coordination	effort needed to move
flow and balance of energy; mood; sense of pleasure	fatigue
muscle tone and strength	compression of discs and nerves
muscular flexibility	adhesions and scarring
posture	muscular tension
range of motion of joints	swelling

Osteopathy

Osteopathic medicine is based on the principle of treating the whole person and facilitating the body's natural ability to heal itself. Osteopathic treatments are based on the theory that the whole body is affected when one part is injured and that improving the flow of blood and nerve function throughout the injured area will help in healing.

Osteopaths may offer treatments that consist of manipulating muscles and bones as well as conventional treatments of drugs and surgery. Osteopathic manipulations have been helpful in promoting recovery from sports injuries and other traumas as well as other causes of neck, back, and joint pain.

Massage

The field of massage contains many disciplines or styles of bodywork. Massage, massage therapy, therapeutic massage, and neuromuscular therapy all refer generally to styles of touch therapy, using the hands to knead, manipulate, and press on the body with various types of motion.

Massage and other bodywork can be helpful after trauma to loosen tight muscles and connective tissue, release muscle spasms, and prevent the formation of scar tissue. Massage also can help reduce swelling and pain by enhancing circulation and lymphatic drainage. Some massage techniques are relaxing and help to reduce stress. Other techniques are invigorating and can elevate your energy level.

For some forms of massage, you'll be asked to undress in private and drape yourself with a sheet or towel so that each part of your body that is being massaged can be uncovered and then redraped. Sometimes lotions or oils are used to improve the flow of the movements and to avoid pulling on body hair. Other forms of massage and bodywork can be performed while you are clothed, provided that you wear loose, comfortable clothing. In most cases, you'll be asked to lie on a padded table. For those who have certain medical conditions that prevent them from being able to lie down, some massage can be done in a chair specially designed to support the head.

Swedish massage is the best-known form of massage. Its practitioners use a variety of strokes—such as smooth, gliding strokes, kneading, and friction—and passive moving and stretching of the body in order to mimic Swedish gymnastics and other forms of exercise. Proponents of Swedish massage believe that it can bring relief from pain and tension and can increase circulation, muscle tone, and the mobility of joints. Because Swedish massage can improve muscle function, it may help those who experience muscle fatigue, weakness, and atrophy resulting from lack of exercise or forced inactivity due to injury.

Thai massage is a technique that combines elements of acupressure, reflexology, and yoga through manual pressure techniques and passive stretching. The recipient wears loose clothing and lies on a mat in order to be able to assume a great variety of body positions while the practitioner applies several techniques. The most expert practitioners of this method are trained in a school located in Wat Pho (Temple of the Reclining Buddha) in Bangkok. This technique can be aggressive, so it may not be appropriate for those who have certain health conditions.

Deep-tissue massage works to release the tension in deep layers of muscles. A therapist may apply slow strokes, strong pressure, or friction with fingers, thumbs, fists, and elbows. This approach is sometimes more effective than Swedish massage for stubborn tension patterns associated with chronic pain. The many types of deep-tissue massage include the Trager Approach and Pfrimmer Deep Muscle Therapy.

Trager, or "Trager psychophysical integration," is a deep-tissue method of massage that blends bodywork with light, gentle movement. Its practitioners believe that this noninvasive method can help release physical and mental tension. The bodywork includes rocking, traction, compression, and exercises to increase range of motion. Exercises called Mentastics are practiced to improve mobility and awareness. The gentleness of these movements prevents increased pain.

Pfrimmer Deep Muscle Therapy uses cross-muscle manipulation to reduce muscular adhesions and stiffness, to improve posture and ease of breathing, to improve circulation of blood and lymphatic fluid, and to reduce entrapment of nerves in soft tissue. Pfrimmer therapy has been helpful in promoting recovery from many conditions, including brain injury, stroke, and other results of trauma.

Movement Techniques for Connective Tissue

The connective tissue below your skin that covers the muscles in your body is called *fascia*. When your body is injured, the fascia absorbs the shock and tightens. As you move, the fascia in other areas of your body tightens in compensation. As a result, you may compromise your posture and coordination, and because movement cannot flow freely, it will take more effort to move.

Several movement techniques are specifically directed toward reducing fascial restrictions, but many other movement techniques described elsewhere in this chapter also affect connective tissue.

Myofascial release is a fascial-release technique often used by osteopaths to relieve pain in muscle tissue. This technique uses gentle, sustained pressure to release restrictions in the fascia and to promote mobility. A practitioner may initially analyze imbalance by observing a patient standing or walking. Then, while the patient reclines, fascia is stretched and the spine decompressed as traction is applied with smooth, gentle strokes. This technique, which helps to normalize the tissue around an injury and helps it to function properly again, has been helpful in rehabilitation from trauma as well as in improving posture.

Rolfing, or "structural integration," is a system of soft-tissue manipulation and movement education designed to improve the body's structure for optimal alignment (posture) and function (movement), using the ideal image of a body organized along a vertical line. This system was developed by an American biochemist, Ida P. Rolf, Ph.D., and became widely known in the 1960s.

Practitioners of this system use firm pressure with their hands, fingers, knuckles, and elbows to relax tight connective tissue and to mobilize joints. Increased mobility allows tissue and joints to return to their normal size and alignment, thus returning balance to the body. Rolfers believe that physical tension patterns and blocked energy that originate from emotional experiences also can be released by these techniques. Rolfers use two approaches to movement. *Rolfing Movement Integration* is designed to train clients to become aware of their posture, to release tension, and to improve their movement habits. *Rolfing Rhythms* is a system of exercise to improve flexibility, muscle tone, and coordination. Although pressure used in Rolfing can be painful, many Rolfers have developed techniques to reduce this discomfort. Some Rolfers also have developed individual methods that incorporate other aspects of manipulation or movement. Any of them could be helpful in treating post-traumatic pain.

Hellerwork is a three-way approach to bodywork—deep-tissue manipulation (including Rolfing as well as massage techniques), movement reeducation, and verbal dialogue. Before developing his own method, Joseph Heller studied Rolfing, Gestalt therapy, Aston Patterning, flotation-tank therapy, and engineering. Hellerwork emphasizes exercises to correct posture, improve common movement patterns, change psychological attitudes, and free self-expression.

Body synergy adds the elements of physical and emotional self-awareness to deep-tissue bodywork, with an additional focus on the healing relationship between practitioner and client. Body synergists believe that this approach can help to change unhealthy attitudes as well as harmful physical patterns.

Aston Patterning is slightly different from other deep-tissue manipulation techniques. It is more gentle than Rolfing and also can include movement education and other forms of bodywork such as massage, myofascial release, and arthrokinetics (joint movements). Its objective is not to aim for linear symmetry of the body; instead, practitioners evaluate their clients' individual needs by exploring specific patterns of movement. After treatment, clients are asked to repeat patterns of movement used for evaluation in order to demonstrate to them what changes have occurred.

Other Forms of Movement Therapy

Craniosacral therapy (CST) is another form of movement therapy. This approach utilizes very gentle manipulations of the bones of the skull and spine to stimulate the nervous system and the membranes and fluid that surround and protect the brain and spinal cord.

When trauma occurs, CST therapists theorize that cerebrospinal fluid loses its normal rhythm. A CST practitioner uses a gentle touch to detect changes in the rhythm of cerebrospinal fluid and works to reduce restrictions and return balance to the movement of these systems in order to allow the body to heal. CST often is used by osteopaths in combination with myofascial-release techniques, and it also is used by physical therapists, massage therapists, and other practitioners. This technique is relaxing, and so gentle that it is safe for most conditions. It can bring relief from headache, dizziness, and pain resulting from trauma.

Visceral manipulation is another gentle manual therapy that is based on the belief that moving the viscera and their connective tissue may increase flexibility of nerves and muscles and raise the level of whole-body function. This technique seems to work very well to release tension and to break distorted patterns that cause pain deep in muscles and nerves.

Zero balancing is a peacefully paced method of movement therapy that combines Eastern and Western approaches to the body to improve healing. A touch at a specific spot becomes a fulcrum around which the body organizes, allowing for as much release and ease as the body can achieve.

Lymph drainage is a manual technique to enhance the flow in the lymph system. By means of a gentle touch, the lymph is encouraged to circulate in a rhythmic way to help the functioning of a blocked area. Techniques used include gently pressing various parts of the body with the palms of the hands and gently moving the fingers to create wavelike movements. Practitioners say that these movements stimulate the circulation of lymph and interstitial fluid, thereby enhancing the functioning of the immune and parasympathetic nervous systems. Swelling may be reduced, toxins eliminated, and pain relieved.

Reflexology is practiced by manually stimulating pressure points on the hands and feet without the use of oils or other implements. The theory is that these pressure points connect to all the organs and glands in the body through the nervous system. There are said to be 7,000 nerve endings in the foot, and stimulating these points may induce relaxation, strengthen organs and glands, and bring relief from pain. Treatments can be performed with a patient fully clothed but barefoot, either lying down or reclining in a seated position. This technique can be a comfortable alternative for those who do not want other parts of their bodies to be touched.

MOVEMENT EDUCATION AND REEDUCATION

Many forms of exercise and movement techniques that were developed for other purposes may be helpful in improving mobility and easing post-traumatic pain, including the Alexander Technique, the Feldenkrais Method, Somatics, Pilates, and the ancient Chinese arts of t'ai chi and chi kung (qigong).

The Alexander Technique

The Alexander Technique (AT) differs from many other techniques because it is a method for learning how to change your body's habits of movement to reduce tension and pain and to improve overall physical functioning. This technique can be taught in small groups or one-on-one and can be tailored to individual physical needs, occupational activities, and interests. This technique uses no physical force.

The Alexander Technique is taught by guiding a student through movement and in stillness with a very light touch, adding verbal observations and visual representations of anatomy to clarify the information. Sometimes certain movements are introduced to break a student's habitual way of moving or to encourage better flexibility or coordination. In a typical lesson, a student will receive this hands-on instruction while standing, sitting, bending, walking, and performing tasks of everyday living such as writing, cooking, cleaning, typing, or lifting. Students who are in chronic pain usually will begin this work lying down, in a position of constructive rest, to help reduce general tension, regain range of motion, and lengthen connective tissue. A student then practices this work between lessons and gradually incorporates the new ways of moving into all activities.

The Feldenkrais Method

The Feldenkrais Method uses repetition of simple, slow movements, without force but with heightened awareness of sensation. The goal of this method is to enhance the function of the neuromuscular system and body-mind connection. Two formats are used: awareness through movement and functional integration.

In *awareness through movement,* verbal instruction is used during group

USING THE ALEXANDER TECHNIQUE TO REDUCE TENSION

Lie on your back on a firm but slightly padded surface placed on the floor. Rest the back of your head on a small paperback book so that your face is parallel to the floor. Put your hands beside your hips, palms down. Bend your knees and place your feet flat, straight in front of your hips.

Ask your whole body to let the surface you are lying on hold your body up. Let go of any tension you can.

Slide your hands along the floor until your arms are outstretched and your fingers are pointing out to the sides. As you do this movement, ask yourself to free your neck and allow the whole back surface of your torso to spread out. Bend your elbows and place the palms of your hands on your ribs. Feel your hands on your body. Let this help you release more tension.

Let your hands sense how your body is moving as you breathe. Let your breathing help you release the tension in your neck.

Slow down. Pay attention to how your body is feeling as it moves. Take it easy, and use less force to move.

classes to guide students slowly through sequences of movements that often are performed sitting or lying on the floor, sitting in a chair, or standing. Sequences of movement generally focus on one part of the body at a time while moving the joints in a flowing sequence. Students are asked to notice the quality of the movement to learn how to perform the pattern of movement with less tension and better coordination.

Functional integration is taught to individuals, with the practitioner using a gentle touch to guide a student gently and slowly through simple movements. Each session can be tailored to the student's condition and level of experience.

In either method, students may practice some of the exercises between sessions, which gives them a sense of control over their healing process. Feldenkrais has helped some students learn to move injured parts of their bodies with less pain by overcoming muscular restrictions, improving posture, and reducing tension.

Somatics

Somatics is a movement system developed by a Feldenkrais practitioner, Thomas Hanna. After an injury, chronic involuntary contractions in the body can cause stiffness, soreness, and "sensory-motor amnesia," a loss of sensation in the muscles and the feeling of how to move them. In Somatics, various slow exercises are practiced, either lying down or in a seated position, to release chronic contractions, to recover sensation of movement, and to improve the flow of movement. Deep breathing is sometimes encouraged. This technique may reduce pain resulting from many forms of trauma.

Pilates

Pilates is a form of exercise developed by Joseph Pilates. Others have created similar forms of exercise based on his principles and methods. Although these exercises can be helpful in the rehabilitation of injuries, Pilates instructors usually are not physical therapists and are not always qualified to work with those who have post-traumatic pain. Look for a qualified practitioner with sufficient experience, and ask for private lessons if you have pain.

These exercises are designed to develop strength, flexibility, posture, and balance. Principles include training with the goals of concentrating on the sensation of movement, lengthening muscles without creating excessive muscle bulk, centering, moving in a slow, flowing way, and breathing in specific patterns throughout the movement. An exercise program can be tailored to an individual's needs, but a student usually works on a mat on the floor as well as with machines. The machines are equipped with springs, cables, bars, straps, and pulleys to facilitate proper alignment of the body in a variety of positions, stretching, and resistance during exercise.

T'ai Chi

T'ai chi ch'uan, also known as t'ai chi, or *taiji,* is an ancient Chinese martial art. However, it also is a form of moving meditation that is practiced as an exercise to enhance physical fitness, health, and relaxation. Generations of teachers have developed several forms, each one a sequence of gentle, flowing movements that are practiced slowly and carefully while adhering to certain principles and philosophies. These principles include moving without the use of excessive muscular force, becoming aware of the movement of energy through your body, maintaining good posture, breathing in a natural way, centering, and grounding. Practicing t'ai chi enhances healing by helping to restore physical, mental, and spiritual balance.

Although t'ai chi may be too challenging for people with certain injuries, it is a safe form of exercise for many others. It can help prevent falls by improving balance and coordination and can help to reduce pain and stiffness, improve circulation, enhance the functioning of the immune system, and reduce stress, fatigue, and depression. It also can help ease certain types of hand, arm, neck, and back pain.

T'ai chi can be practiced by partners in a sparring game called "push-hands." Push-hands may not be advisable for many of those who are still healing from post-traumatic pain, except in its most gentle, noncompetitive form.

Chi Kung (Qigong)

Chi kung, or *qigong,* is a Chinese form of exercise thought to predate t'ai chi by several thousand years. Most forms of chi kung are easier to learn than t'ai chi and may be more easily practiced by those who have pain.

This method is not a martial art—its movements have no applications for fighting or self-defense—but it shares many of the benefits and principles of t'ai chi, such as conforming to Chinese philosophy of the laws of balance and harmony and the concept of moving energy by focusing the mind.

There are thousands of forms of chi kung. A chi kung expert may be able to designate which exercises may enhance the function of certain organs and which exercises would be helpful to heal from trauma. Some forms of chi kung are short, simple movement sequences. Each movement is designed to help balance the body's energy (*chi,* or *qi*), and to enhance the flow of energy through the energy channels, or meridians, in order to strengthen the internal organs and other systems. Each exercise is practiced slowly in a flowing pattern while breathing freely and continually in a specific pattern. The best results in terms of improved health, fitness, and well-being are gained when exercises are practiced daily.

Certain forms of chi kung consist of holding postures and focusing on breathing patterns, centering, grounding, and the flow of energy. Other forms of chi kung involve the use of meditation on images and energy; for example, "external chi kung" concentrates on the transfer of energy by a chi kung master to a patient to enhance healing.

ENERGETIC HEALING THERAPIES

This category of bodywork includes techniques that are theorized to affect the flow of energy in or near the body—the energy that is known as life force, *chi, qi, prana,* and electric, magnetic, and electromagnetic fields, as well as many other names. Some of these techniques also use some of the therapies described above.

Shiatsu

The Japanese form of manual therapy called shiatsu uses principles of acupressure, a Chinese manual therapy. However, shiatsu also incorporates some techniques from Western massage. Based on the belief that trauma can disrupt the body's flow of energy, the objectives of shiatsu are to unblock and balance the flow of energy throughout the body by stimulating a series of specific points situated on meridians (lines or pathways of energy) along the body. Stimulating these points can have either a toning (strengthening) or sedating (weakening) effect, depending upon what is needed.

Treatments are given while the client lies down or sits, fully clothed in loose, lightweight clothing. Shiatsu has been useful in relieving nausea, postoperative pain, and insomnia.

Tuina

Tuina is a Chinese method of therapeutic massage that is designed with principles of Chinese medicine. Its goal is to relieve pain and to improve health by activating the body's energy (*chi,* or *qi*). Techniques include touching some pressure points as well as other forms of manipulation.

A CASE IN POINT: USING SEVERAL BODYWORK TECHNIQUES TO HEAL

Jackie has been the unlucky victim of three automobile accidents during the past eight years. Then, while she was trying to recover from her last accident, she slipped on a patch of ice and landed hard on her back.

Medical doctors have diagnosed her at various times with lumbosacral strain, nerve damage, herniated discs, arthritis, costochondritis, fibromyalgia, and chronic fatigue. For years she has had chronic back pain, tightness and weakness in her chest and arms, and extreme general fatigue. For quite a while she was disabled; she could not work, lift a coffee cup, open a door, drive a car, or hold a telephone receiver or a book. She spent most of her days and nights sleeping, and she became fearful of further injury. She was depressed and easily angered.

During the past eight years, Jackie has assembled a team of doctors and alternative-treatment practitioners and teachers who have helped her recover to a great degree.

After her first accident, which was very serious, she saw a neurologist and internist, who gave her some helpful medications. She also saw a psychiatrist, who prescribed a daily pattern of rest and activity. The program was a schedule for getting up and being active for two hours, then sleeping or resting for two hours, in a pattern repeated throughout the day. This helped her to regulate her symptoms.

Jackie also worked with a Feldenkrais practitioner who helped her to increase her flexibility and energy level and decrease her pain. Later, her psychiatrist referred her to the author so that she could learn the Alexander Technique. An individual exercise program was developed for her, using the principles of the Alexander Technique, and she has continued to work with this program, modifying it as her health has progressed. This program consists of several strategies:

- Receiving the hands-on work of the Alexander Technique to reduce pressure and chronic tension in her body.
- Practicing very gentle movement exercises at certain intervals during the day, some of which consist of everyday movements done in new ways, with a very slow progression to build flexibility and strength.

For example, she began by lifting a paper plate from a table by bending her knees, then bending her elbows to lift the plate. After two months, a small weight (an audiocassette tape) was added to the plate; then more and more weight was added over a period of time. Then she began carrying the weighted plate across the room.

- Using constructive rest positions (sitting and lying down) periodically throughout the day.
- Learning good body mechanics.
- Learning to take a gentler, more relaxed approach to movement.
- Learning to bear emotional stress without letting it affect her body so much.

After Jackie had been practicing the Alexander Technique for two years, this author suggested that she see a physical therapist for soft-tissue manipulation. That therapist performed myofascial-release and craniosacral-release techniques that seemed to help reduce restrictions in her nerves and muscles and improve her flexibility.

As her body gained coordination, we were able to add chi kung exercises to her program. These she enjoyed so much that she gradually replaced some of the other exercises she was doing. Chi kung improved her movement flow, grounding, balance, level of relaxation, and pleasure.

Gradually, Jackie developed skills that helped her regain control of her body. She has had periods of time when she has no pain. When she does experience pain and stiffness from more activity than her body can handle, she knows how to loosen herself through movement and relaxation. Now she can drive, lift and carry dishes, open doors, talk on the telephone, lift books, and work at her desk a couple of hours each day.

Watsu

Watsu is a form of bodywork that is practiced in water that is just below body temperature. It combines elements of shiatsu and yoga and is very helpful in releasing tension and improving the flow of energy.

Therapeutic Touch

One of the safest, least invasive techniques available is therapeutic touch. This method was developed by a nurse and is practiced by many nurses as part of their nurturing routines. To clear, direct, and modulate the flow of energy in a client, practitioners hold their hands three to six inches above a patient's body in order to detect disturbances in the energy flow such as sluggishness, congestion, or excessive amounts of energy. Slow, wavelike motions of the hands are used in order to, in theory, move, clear, and balance the client's field of energy.

Therapeutic touch can be administered preoperatively to induce relaxation and reduce anxiety, and postoperatively to reduce pain.

Reiki

Reiki means "universal life-force energy." A practitioner places his or her hands in certain positions on or near a recipient's body in order to, in theory, allow the universal life-force energy to flow. The positions usually begin at the crown of the recipient's head and move toward the feet. No massage is performed.

Reiki practitioners believe that areas of the body's energy field become blocked or weakened by injury or illness and that the flow of energy that occurs during a Reiki session can promote healing of physical injuries and illness as well as mental and emotional illness. They believe that by clearing the underlying (karmic) causes of a problem, a client may return to health and harmony. Reiki stimulates a relaxation response, and after a session, a recipient usually feels less pain and discomfort, more peaceful, and more content.

AWARENESS TRAINING

Biofeedback, hypnotherapy, and the many forms of meditation, including yoga, can help you to achieve better control over your body. Yoga is discussed in detail in Chapter 17.

Biofeedback

Biofeedback is a system that uses instruments to provide information about the body, such as its physical reactions to stress, in order to make it possible to control physical processes that are usually involuntary. Its objectives are to learn to relax, to reduce pain, and to reduce other symptoms of stress.

By means of electrical sensors placed on the skin, biofeedback instruments can be used to monitor changes in temperature, muscular activity, electrodermal activity, heart rate, brain waves, and respiration. By receiving feedback in the form of sound or electrical signals, you can learn to warm cold hands, reduce your heart rate, and slow your breathing.

Meditation

The object of meditation is to center yourself and bring balance and unity to your mind, body, and emotions. As you meditate, the chatter of everyday thoughts recedes and you become more peaceful. The relaxation you achieve can help reduce pain and anxiety and improve your breathing and ease of movement. Meditation often improves spiritual understanding and empathy and could help you to accept your own condition as well as that of others.

A vast number of types of meditation are available, all of them tools for relaxation, healing, and spiritual growth. Any one of them could be useful in the management of pain and stress. Most forms include sitting upright on a cushion, bench, or chair and focusing your mind on something specific. For example:

- Count to ten over and over again.
- Notice the sensation of your breath in your nostrils.
- Look at or visualize an image.
- Be aware—simply sit still and pay attention to what you are experiencing physically, mentally, and emotionally in the present moment.
- Focus on a sound, either an external sound or one mentally repeated.

Other meditation styles include movement, either structured or improvised, including walking and dancing. The many styles of meditation include transcendental meditation (TM), Zen and other forms of Buddhist meditation, Christian meditation, yoga, mindfulness, Sufism, t'ai chi, and authentic movement.

Hypnotherapy

Hypnotherapy is used to induce relaxation through the special state of sleeping called a hypnotic trance. To achieve this, a patient is instructed with commands repeated in a soothing, monotonous voice to relax parts of the body and to focus on breathing, thereby moving attention inward and away from the environment. In this state, a patient has a heightened receptivity to suggestion.

Hypnotherapy has helped many people learn to relax and cope with pain. However, hypnosis is not safe for everyone, so if you would like to try this therapy, be sure to check with a mental-health professional first.

YOUR OWN TREATMENT

When you and your doctors decide that it is safe to add complementary therapies or movement to your treatment, you can choose from a great variety of bodywork techniques. For a more comprehensive description and discussion of each technique described in this chapter, visit the Web site of *The Gale Encyclopedia of Alternative Medicine.* You'll also find other sources in "Suggested Readings" and "Helpful Web Sites and Organizations."

You may discover that there are many bodywork techniques that could help you. However, the location of practitioners or teachers in your community may determine whom you can see and how often. A series of treatments or lessons on a regular schedule is preferable.

EVALUATING YOUR EXPERIENCE

After your first treatment or lesson, ask yourself:

- Did I feel safe? Was the practitioner or teacher careful not to injure me?
- Was the teacher sufficiently aware of my physical limitations and pain to administer the proper treatment?

- Did the practitioner demonstrate a high level of skill?
- Did I enjoy the session?
- Did I feel better, worse, or the same afterward? If I had pain afterward, did the pain go away? Did I later feel better than before the treatment? (Sometimes you have to feel a little worse for a while before you begin to feel better.)

AFTER A TREATMENT or a new experience, give yourself time to experience the changes that have occurred in your body and to sense how they are influencing your movement. Ask your practitioner what is reasonable to expect following a treatment, and ask for advice about your activity following treatment.

Ask for help. Experiment. Trust your body's inner knowledge. Take your time, but decide to heal. Move on with your life.

SUGGESTED READINGS

"The Alexander Technique: Application to Medical Rehabilitation and Published Research." Available through the North American Society of Teachers of the Alexander Technique: 1-800-473-0620.

Burton Goldberg Group. "Craniosacral Therapy," in *Alternative Medicine: The Definitive Guide.* Puyallup, WA: Future Medicine Publishing, Inc., 1993.

Feldenkrais, Moshe. *Awareness Through Movement: Health Exercises for Personal Growth.* New York: Harper & Row, 1972, 1977.

Kodish, Bruce I., Ph.D. *Back Pain Solutions: How to Help Yourself with Posture-Movement Therapy and Education.* Pasadena, CA: Extensional Publishing, 2001.

Krapp, K., Longe, J.L., eds. *The Gale Encyclopedia of Alternative Medicine.* Farmington Hills, MI: The Gale Group, 2000.

MacDonald, Glynn. *The Complete Illustrated Guide to the Alexander Technique: A Practical Program for Health, Poise, and Fitness.* Shaftesbury, Dorset; Boston, MA; Melbourne, Victoria: Element Books, 1998.

McFarlane, Stewart. *The Complete Book of T'ai Chi.* New York: DK Publishing, 1997.

Ramsey, Susan M., PT, MA. "Holistic Manual Therapy Techniques," in *Complementary and Alternative Therapies in Primary Care,* vol. 24, no. 4, December 1997.

Rolf, Ida. P. *Rolfing: Reestablishing the Natural Alignment and Structural Integration of the Human Body for Vitality and Well-Being.* Rochester, VT: Healing Arts Press, 1989.

Sarno, John E. *Healing Back Pain: The Mind-Body Connection.* New York: Warner Books, 1991.

Weintraub, William. *Tendon and Ligament Healing: A New Approach Through Manual Therapy.* Berkeley, CA: North Atlantic Books, 1999.

Wright, S.M. "The use of therapeutic touch in the management of pain," *Reviews Registry, enl, Complementary Medicine Program,* http://registry.ummc.umaryland.edu/RIS/RISWEB.ISA., Vol. 22, Issue 3, 1987, p. 705.

HELPFUL WEB SITES AND ORGANIZATIONS

Alexander Technique International
1692 Massachusetts Ave., 3rd Floor
Cambridge, MA 02138
Telephone: 888-321-0856
http://www.ati-net.com

American Board of Hypnotherapy
16842 Von Karman Avenue, Suite 476
Irvine, CA 92714
http://www.hypnosis.com

American Massage Therapy Association
http://www.amtamassage.org

American Osteopathic Association
142 East Ontario St.
Chicago, IL 60611
Telephone: 312-280-5800
http://www.aoa-net.org

The American Physical Therapy Association
1111 N. Fairfax St.
Alexandria, VA 22314
Telephone: 800-999-2782
http://www.apta.org

The Biofeedback Network
On-Line Biofeedback Resources
http://www.biofeedback.net

The Feldenkrais Guild of North America
706 Ellsworth St.
P.O. Box 478
Albany, OR 97321-0143
Telephone: 800-775-2118
http://www.feldenkrais.com

Gale Encyclopedia of Alternative Medicine
http://www.gale.com

The International Association of Reiki Professionals
P.O. Box 481
Winchester, MA 01890
http://www.iarp.org

The Rolf Institute of Structural Integration
Telephone: 800-530-8875
http://www.rolf.org

The Upledger Institute, Inc.
11211 Prosperity Farms Road
Palm Beach Gardens, FL 33410
Telephone: 800-233-5330
http://www.upledger.com

For information on craniosacral therapy.

13

Eat Better to Feel Better

GLORIA HORWITZ, M.S.

No foods can eliminate pain, but some foods can help you be a more energetic, focused, and contented person. The right foods can help you manage your mood, lower your awareness of pain, and give you the energy you need to live your life to its fullest.

Too often, the stresses caused by trauma and the process of recovery lead to disturbances in eating behavior. Those disturbances create additional stress, perpetuating the cycle of metabolic dysfunction. Nutritional therapy can dramatically reduce post-traumatic pain and stress, and can help you feel better, both physically and mentally. When you feel better about yourself and what you're doing in life, you'll focus on your accomplishments and your recreational activities rather than on your pain.

CRAVINGS

It's common knowledge that prolonged stress is often accompanied by a gain in weight, and researchers have documented a link between pain, stress, and chemicals in our bodies that can cause us to put on weight.

Stress stimulates the breakdown of serotonin, a neurotransmitter located in the brain that regulates mood and appetite. The breakdown of serotonin triggers the adrenal glands to stimulate the production of a nerve chemical in the brain called neuropeptide Y (NPY). As the level of serotonin falls and the level of NPY rises, cravings increase for carbohydrates—especially sweets.

Continued consumption of sweets causes the level of insulin to rise and plummet very quickly, producing feelings that range from euphoria to depression: One minute after you eat a candy bar you feel energized, and ten minutes later all that energy is gone. Low energy causes you to focus more on your pain and stress, both of which further drain your energy.

In this chapter, you'll meet patients who have learned to use nutritional therapy to ease their post-traumatic stress and pain. You'll learn about several types of eating imbalances, and you'll learn some strategies to bring your own eating habits into balance.

EATING PATTERNS

One day, a patient named Roberta came into my office complaining of persistent pain in her knees and back after being injured in an automobile accident a year earlier. Despite extensive medical care, she still could not cope with her post-traumatic pain.

Roberta confessed that she had been consuming large amounts of sugar to comfort herself. As a result, she had gained thirty pounds since her accident. At 5' 1" in height, Roberta had added more weight than her frame could comfortably support, putting more pressure on her knees and back. This weight gain also had affected her mood; she was mildly depressed, because every time she looked in a mirror she could see how her body had ballooned since her accident.

At our first meeting, Roberta and I discussed an eating plan that would help her reach two goals. The first would be to shed those thirty pounds. The second goal would be to find a satisfying and gratifying way to lose this weight so that she would change her focus from "living to eat" to "eating to live." I didn't want to exile Roberta to a land of deprivation and starvation; I wanted her to be able to feel positive about her progress without feeling hungry.

One of our strategies was to reduce her post-traumatic stress and depression. We began by identifying her "eating pattern," a concept I developed through my sixteen years' experience with weight loss and stress management.

If you can give it a name, you can win the game. My research has shown that identifying your eating pattern enables you to focus on your individual food needs. The following are four typical eating patterns that I have found to be most common; you may recognize yourself in more than one category.

Grazers eat all day long, never sitting down to a meal. They prefer snacking and eating out of boxes, bags, and containers. Grazers tend to eat standing up or while they talk on the telephone. They like finger food of any kind. A grazer is always tasting and testing foods throughout the cooking process, perhaps eating half of the cookies while they're cooling on the cookie sheet. Grazers consume large quantities of any kind of snack, including the low-fat kind.

Constant eaters have a lot in common with grazers, but they eat regular meals as well as between-meal snacks. Constant eaters think that they don't have time to eat, yet they eat all the time. Unlike grazers, a constant eater never stops eating.

Plate-cleaners think that they must finish everything in front of them. When they were children, their parents probably ordered them to clean their plates.

Justifiers eat nothing all day long so that they can eat anything they want all night: They starve all day so that they can stuff all night. They consume most of their food after 6 P.M. No one sees them eat.

An Eating Plan for a Grazer

It was easy to identify Roberta as a grazer. All day long, she grazed on sugary sweets such as cookies, candy, ice cream, and frozen yogurt. The first step for Roberta was to recognize and accept that she was a mindless eater of sugar. I asked her to begin marking off the amount of food she consumed on the outside of each container, and she was startled when she became aware of the quantity of food she was consuming. She realized that she tended to almost unconsciously graze while watching TV, talking on the phone, or engaging in other activities.

The next step was for Roberta to recognize and use the concept of closure—closure of eating. She had to decide what she was going to eat, and how much, so that she had a place to stop and close each grazing session. For example, Roberta learned to count out sixteen jelly beans, put them on a plate, remind herself that she had chosen sixteen, and decide how long she wanted to take to eat them.

The first time Roberta tried this, she ate all sixteen jelly beans in less than a minute. I suggested that the next time she ate the jelly beans she take the sixteen and divide them into two servings of eight. She put those servings into little plastic bags. This allowed her to snack more frequently without increasing the volume. The next step was to divide the jelly beans among four bags. This slowed down her intake of food as well as her sugar dependency. It also allowed her to continue to use jelly beans as a comfort food in order to cope with her post-traumatic pain without the damaging results of weight gain.

In one month, by using the closure concept for all of her snacking, Roberta dropped eight pounds. She was delighted with herself, and losing those eight pounds motivated her to continue her weight-loss program.

The key to Roberta's success was planning: Planning is stronger than willpower. Carbohydrate snacks, chosen in moderation, can help any grazer who feels jittery or who has trouble focusing. Good choices of snacks include sixteen jelly beans, six graham crackers, one cup of cereal without milk, or an apple cut into several slices so that it looks like more.

Roberta was able to change the way she thinks, not just the way she eats. This thinking enabled her to lose the next ten pounds. I suggested that she reward herself by going out and spending as much time as possible shopping for a gift for herself that was not food-related—jewelry, a scarf, a book, perfume, or anything else that she could enjoy as a reminder of her success. Roberta bought herself a beautiful pair of earrings, but she received a gift more precious than any piece of jewelry: She realized that during all this time she hadn't focused on her post-traumatic pain because she was focusing on her new possibilities.

When we mollify ourselves with comfort foods, few of us ever crave steak or grilled-cheese sandwiches. Instead, we want the instant gratification of sweet or salty things that come out of a box or a bag—cookies, candy, cake, pretzels, chips, and nuts. But the comfort we find in these sugary or salty foods lasts only a moment. This results in a tendency to overeat, moment after moment, on comfort foods; this increases our weight, which increases our stress level, which can increase our pain, especially if we have gained more weight than our bones can easily carry.

Salt and sugar are the universal tranquilizers: They never answer you back, never give you a hard time, and never disappoint you—until you try to stand up. Don't give up! Others have learned how and what to eat to slim down and feel better despite their pain, and so can you.

An Eating Plan for a Constant Eater

The day that Mark entered my office for the first time, he had a long face. He felt stressed and upset about the new lifestyle he had been forced to adopt as a result of a skiing accident. He was in pain, and he had difficulty walking and balancing. Even more than skiing, Mark missed his regular rounds of golf. He was in mourning for his lost athleticism.

As a result of having been idle, Mark had became a constant eater. During the past year, he had put on fifty pounds, most of it in his abdomen. For men, weight gain in the stomach area poses a serious health threat: It can lead to elevated cholesterol, high blood pressure, diabetes, heart disease, and other health problems.

It occurred to me that he and I could help each other. I had recently returned from a week of golf camp (actually, to me it had felt like boot camp). Although I had been told that when I left camp I would have a golf swing, that golf swing was still undeveloped by the time I met Mark. I struck a deal with Mark: I would help him lose weight and deal with his constant eating, while helping him reduce his post-traumatic pain. In return, I asked if he would help me with my golf swing. Although Mark was not able to play golf, he was more than capable of instructing me, particularly since he had a handicap of five. We shook on it. I knew I was in good hands.

I told Mark that once he lost fifty pounds, he would be able to return to the golf course to play. He might not be able to play as long or as often as before his accident, but play he would. When I asked Mark if he thought that his expanding middle might be getting in the way of his golf swing, as well as contributing to his post-traumatic pain, he sheepishly nodded in the affirmative.

The first thing that Mark and I discussed was his regular fare on a typical day. He agreed to keep a ledger of what he consumed at breakfast, mid-morning, lunch, mid-afternoon, before dinner, dinner, after dinner, and for bedtime snacks; that's how often he was eating.

Mark's ledger showed that his meals consisted mostly of buttery, fatty foods such as lunch meats, cheeses, fast-food snacks, and leftovers such as macaroni and cheese. He loved McDonald's and Burger King and would almost inhale the food so quickly that he hardly realized that he was eating. Only when I asked him to save the bag from the french fries did he realize that not only was he eating fatty french fries, but he was also consuming the largest portion available.

Fatty foods slow the digestive process, causing sluggishness and increasing tiredness and depression. Protein-rich foods such as fish, chicken, and meat were needed to add more tyrosine, an amino acid, to Mark's diet. Tyrosine encourages the production of two chemicals in the brain, dopamine and norepinephrine, which enhance mental ability and stimulate a sense of well-being. Foods rich in protein also take longer to digest, and once Mark began to add these to his daily diet, he began to feel fuller for longer periods of time.

Mark discovered that he had actually lost the ability to differentiate between feeling full and feeling stuffed. I wanted Mark to eat more slowly so that he could learn to recognize sooner when he was full. It takes twenty minutes to digest food and for your nerves to send a message to your brain that you are satisfied and full. Mark became conscious of the difference between being full and being stuffed by learning to eat more slowly and to take at least twenty minutes (using an oven timer) to complete each meal. He was amazed at the pleasure he felt from taking additional time to eat.

Weight loss truly begins in the head. Mark understood this, but he complained that food was the only comfort he could rely on to help him deal with his post-traumatic pain and stress throughout the day. He understood that he was using food as pain medication to deal with his new life. But he was at a loss as to how to change his behavior.

To change his choice of foods, we began with breakfast. Mark liked a big breakfast of fruit and cereal together with eggs, bacon, and toast. First I asked him to exchange his white-flour toast for whole-wheat or rye. We decided to divide his breakfast into two meals: His first breakfast would consist of toast, bacon, and cereal or eggs. His second breakfast, which was to be finished by mid-morning, was fruit—an apple, orange, or grapefruit.

TIPS TO SLOW DOWN AND ENJOY A LEISURELY MEAL

- Cut your food into small pieces.
- Sip some water as you eat.
- Put down your fork between bites.
- Have some conversation during your meal.
- If possible, find a dining companion who eats more slowly than you do.

Mark's next step was to apply time management to food: He was to eat lunch no later than four hours after his first breakfast. His new lunches consisted of protein foods such as fish, chicken, or meat in a salad or on a sandwich, to be consumed within a twenty-minute period.

Another challenge for Mark was to avoid eating a huge volume of food while he was deciding what to eat for his next meal. Simply put, he had to learn the three Ws: "What, when, and where am I going to eat?" He needed to predetermine what he was going to eat before each meal; this would help him stick to his plan without overeating. If he felt ravenous before lunch, he would eat a sliced apple.

Within two weeks, Mark moved his belt buckle over a notch, and he could bend over to tie his shoes more easily. He was encouraged and amazed that his hunger and his constant need to eat were abating. At last he felt satisfied after a meal, and he noticed that with less fat on his body, he was feeling less pain.

Mark learned firsthand that planning is stronger than willpower. Although it took him about twenty weeks to drop fifty pounds, it took me only ten weeks to improve my golf swing. We both became winners.

An Eating Plan for a Plate-Cleaner

Did your mother or grandmother always tell you to finish what's on your plate or to "think of the starving children of the world"? Now that you can choose the size of your portions, fill your plate consciously and learn to know when you are satisfied.

Fred is a policeman whose eating habits were changed by trauma. One afternoon while he was off duty, he saw a robbery taking place at a convenience store. His training automatically kicked into gear, and he tackled the robber and knocked him to the ground. He saved the lives of the cashiers and customers, but the robber fired his gun before he could be subdued and shot Fred in the leg. This injury caused permanent damage and persistent pain in Fred's leg.

Fred became confined to a desk job, and after several surgeries and extensive physical therapy, he realized that his role as a policeman was forever altered. Unhappy and restless, he consoled himself with food. Even before his accident, Fred had been a plate-cleaner; now he heaped piles of food onto his plate and still felt that he had to finish every morsel. He had become out of shape, out of breath, and out of control in his eating habits. When he entered my office, he was depressed, bitter, lethargic, angry, in pain, and ashamed of himself.

After talking with Fred, I realized that the problem wasn't what he was eating—it was how much. The plan to help him lose weight, reduce his pain, and recover his sense of self-esteem would require him to learn new eating techniques. He would always be a plate-cleaner, but he could put less food on his plate. Then he could finish his meal just as he always did, without putting on the pounds.

Fred was not happy about the prospect of eating less. I suggested that he put the usual amount of food on his plate, divide it in half, and place it on two plates. Then he was to wait at least seven minutes after finishing plate one before beginning plate two. To Fred, seven minutes seemed like an eternity. However, much to his amazement, after learning to wait seven minutes, he found that he did not always want the entire amount of food on plate number two. If he did eat all of it, he felt stuffed and uncomfortable.

Next, Fred learned to combine his two plates of food into a lesser volume on one plate. However, he always knew that once he did this, he could finish that plate of food.

Fred was still a plate-cleaner, but now he ate less. The pounds dropped off easily, and Fred began to like himself better. He was less lethargic and had more mobility. The stress on his leg was reduced. His pain lessened, too. As he started to feel better, he was able to walk longer distances, which also helped him to lose weight, strengthen the muscles in his leg, and manage his pain.

An Eating Plan for a Justifier

Unlike grazers, constant eaters, and plate-cleaners, justifiers starve all day to feel entitled to eat anything and everything all night.

This was Sara's problem. She had been an obese child and an obese teenager, and she had become an obese adult. Her obesity caused chronic back pain and made her depressed. Sara had tried every quick-fix weight-loss plan, from high-protein to low-carbohydrate diets; she had counted points and counted calories. Nothing worked. Sara had yet to deal with the fact that she was feeding the psychological pain of being an unhappy, obese child. She also was unaware of her pattern of eating.

Sara's enjoyment of food and the comfort it gave her, both physically and psychologically, was manifested only at night when she was alone. The first ten minutes after she arrived home became a dangerous time for her.

Her coworkers never saw her eat. All day long, Sara didn't eat; she had no hunger because she ate all night. Not eating all day made her feel self-righteous and entitled to eat all night when she got home. To assuage her loneliness and her pain, she ate mindlessly.

Surprisingly, Sara admitted that she consumed all of this food in every room of her apartment *except* the kitchen. She ate while she watched television. She ate while she talked on the phone. She ate in bed. Sara even told me, with great embarrassment, that she kept a small refrigerator in her bedroom so that she wouldn't have to travel far for a snack. For Sara, food had become a security blanket.

The first priority was to help Sara become aware of her behavior. I asked her to identify and list all the foods that she consumed throughout the night, numbering them in the order of her favorite foods. We then picked the top ten choices, with the goal of eliminating all others. Sara was very reluctant to give up so many of her comfort foods, but she agreed to try.

Next Sara agreed to sit down, either at the kitchen table or the dining table, for all of her meals. We started by scheduling breakfast. Lunch also became mandatory, and she was permitted to have a snack of fruit on her way home from work. Sara also was instructed to set the table at which she would be dining as soon as she arrived home. While deciding her dinner choice, she was allowed to eat an additional fruit that she cut into slices. She was learning where to eat, when to eat, and how to allocate realistic proportions.

In the beginning, time restrictions were set. Sara was permitted to eat her dinner and snacks from 7:00 P.M. to 11:00 P.M., but always at the table. The next big hurdle was to remove the refrigerator from her bedroom: The new rule was that no food or drink was to be allowed in there. She bravely agreed.

Sara used me as a coach to check in with her every week and to hold her responsible for her progress. She began to lose two pounds a week. She couldn't believe it! Every diet she had tried before had only made her suffer more. She was thrilled that she had begun to conquer her constant nighttime eating.

Sara began to have lunch with coworkers at her office. As she learned to manage her eating times, she began to lose body fat. This decreased her back pain and motivated her to continue her plan. She has been working at her plan for a year, and now there is considerably less of Sara. She spends more time participating in social activities that do not revolve around food, and she is building her social calendar. She is much happier, and she has less pain.

STRESS

How does stress cause pain? You've heard these phrases: "He's on my back about work every day." "She's a pain in the neck." "I'm going to have to shoulder the responsibility." "Just grit your teeth and do it." "I can't stomach the situation." No wonder we're in pain! But you can do something about it.

First, notice where your pain is located. Once you recognize your pains, you'll be better able to deal with them. The following are some physical problems that often result from post-traumatic pain and stress:

- back pain.
- leg and joint pain.
- teeth-grinding.
- indigestion.
- migraine headaches.
- frequent colds and flu.

- a tendency to be accident-prone, which causes broken bones and injury to soft tissues.
- sapped energy.

There is no magic recipe to curb the effects of stress, but you can ease your pain by giving your body the nutrients it needs for optimal health and healing. The following are a few foods that provide extra benefits:

- Whole-grain breads help speed the amino acid tryptophan to the brain. There, tryptophan raises levels of serotonin, which is thought to act as a sedative.
- Oranges are rich in potassium, an electrolyte that conducts nerve impulses and helps the brain's neurotransmitters to work properly.
- Fish is rich in B vitamins, as are potatoes and beef. Insufficient quantities of these vitamins have been associated with anxiety, irritability, and mood swings.
- Rice is rich in thiamine. Some researchers have linked deficiency of thiamine to depression. You also can get the thiamine you need from pork, fish, beans, enriched breads and cereals, and sunflower seeds.
- Spinach and other green vegetables such as Swiss chard and artichokes are loaded with magnesium, a mineral crucial to the body's general defense against stress. Wheat germ, peanuts, soybeans, and bananas are other excellent sources of magnesium.

Choosing some of these foods on a daily basis will boost your energy, elevate your mood, reduce stress, and allow you to be more active.

CREATE YOUR OWN EATING PLAN

To use food to make yourself feel better, you must identify your personal eating type. Are you a grazer, a constant eater, a plate-cleaner, or a justifier? Like Roberta, Fred, Mark, and Sara, you can use strategies to make your plan a success. Once you take the first step, you'll find it possible to become healthier and slimmer and to reduce your pain.

Numerous studies have confirmed that our daily intake of the right foods relaxes every aspect of our bodies, from brain waves to muscle tension. Even when we are focused on our pain and feeling keyed up and jittery, we can use food—in moderation—as a way to calm down and reduce the pain. Time management of eating regulates blood sugar and will help you to be more relaxed.

Let food have its calming effect on you. Discover which foods are best for you in times of stress, and live your plan.

14

Herbal Therapy for Chronic Pain

SHARON L. KOLASINSKI, M.D.

The flowers, leaves, and roots of plants have been used for thousands of years by humans seeking an improvement in the quality of their daily lives. A 5,300-year-old Ice Man discovered in the Swiss Alps was found to have the woody fruit of a bracket fungus, known to have antibiotic and laxative properties, among his personal effects. Many cultures have incorporated indigenous herbs into traditional ceremonial, religious, and medical practices because of their pharmacological properties. Some of these uses remain a part of the modern practice of, for instance, Chinese or Ayurvedic medicine. Some herbs are being newly discovered by consumers as they survey the shelves of local natural-products retailers. Out of cultural or historical context, a consumer may pick up a bottle of an herb extract and wonder, "Will this help me feel better?" In this chapter, a number of aspects of using herbal medicines for treatment of chronic pain will be addressed.

It is important to remember throughout this discussion, however, that herbal treatments often involve the use of biologically active ingredients. This means that herbal treatments produce effects in the human body that can be physiologically and functionally significant. After all, plant extracts have been used by humans for millennia because they have actual, and not just imagined, effects. Sometimes this means that the herbs will be of benefit in treating the condition for which they are intended. Sometimes this means that they will have important, but perhaps unintended and adverse, side effects. Therefore, herbal treatments need to be thought of like any other medications. Due consideration for and attention to the correct dose, the timing of doses, potential for side effects, and possible interactions with other medications should be given.

Furthermore, no single herbal treatment, just as no single prescription drug, is likely to relieve all pain. Taking more and more herbal medicines, vitamins, or other supplements does not necessarily mean more and more pain relief. This is illustrated by a patient who came to me with chronic, debilitating pain, osteoarthritis, and fibromyalgia. Her pain had started twelve years earlier after a fall. She developed chronic low back pain and, later, chest pain, knee pain, and then generalized leg pain. As she became increasingly disabled by her pain, she sought care from a variety of alternative providers. Each "prescribed" what he or she felt to be appropriate treatment, and the patient simply added each suggestion to the others. She arrived at her first visit to my office with a list of fifty-seven different vitamins, minerals, and herbs that she was taking, with no more pain relief than when she was taking none of them. This example illustrates that the use of herbal medications should be put in the context of the overall pain-management plan. Herbal medications are not a substitute for other components of the management plan like exercise, coping skills, or assistive devices. With improvement in her outlook and sense of self-efficacy, an enhanced exercise program, and a total knee replacement, my patient was able to reduce her intake of over-the-counter supplements by 80 percent. Attention to aspects of her overall care, not just the number of pills containing natural "cures," proved to be the most helpful approach.

WHAT'S IN THE BOTTLE?

Herbal medicines are increasingly one of the options chosen by patients in pain. The availability of herbal preparations to the consumer was enhanced by the passage of the 1994 Dietary Supplement and Health Education Act. This legislation permitted herbal medicines to be classified as "botanicals" rather than as drugs. This, in turn, allowed manufacturers to market them as "dietary supplements" without being subject to the rigorous scientific evaluation that helps ensure the safety and effectiveness of prescription drugs. It is important to remember that, despite being available in almost every corner drugstore, not to mention on thousands of Internet sites, over-the-counter herbal products are not regulated in the same way that prescription medicines are. This means consumers do not have the same assurance about what is in the bottle in terms of actual ingredients, their purity, their potency, or whether the preparation works and, if so, how and why it works. This has had several consequences.

First, consumers cannot be completely sure of what they are getting when they buy over-the-counter herbal drugs. Medical investigation into herbal medicines has been hampered as well. Researchers often do not know what the active ingredient in an herbal preparation is. Furthermore, even when one product is tested, conclusions about all products containing the supposed active ingredient may be inappropriate because over-the-counter products may vary so widely in what they actually contain. Finally, some over-the-counter preparations have been adulterated during the manufacturing process, with devastating consequences. One weight-loss botanical, a Chinese herbal preparation made with *Stephania tetrandra,* for instance, is now known to have been contaminated with *Aristolochia fangchi,* an herb that led to kidney failure early on in some who took it and is now leading to cancer in others.

In choosing herbal medicine, what guidelines can be followed to ensure that they are used so that they are as effective and as safe as possible? It is probably best to choose manufacturers with a national reputation. Even some pharmaceutical companies are now in the natural-products business, selling herbal preparations over the counter under well-known drug-company names. If possible, investigate whether or not independent laboratory testing of brands has occurred. This information may be available in popular publications such as *Consumer Reports.* Additional information is available on a variety of Internet sites. (See "Helpful Web Sites" on page 229.) In particular, it is useful to know if testing has confirmed the presence of the presumed active ingredient and how much is present in a particular brand. Consumers should always read the label for the list of ingredients. Potential buyers should avoid products that do not have labeling in a language that they understand. Caution should be used in obtaining herbal preparations from alternative providers who mix the preparations themselves. For ready-to-use treatments, consumers should never exceed the manufacturer's recommended dose; it may be the only available guideline for the appropriate dose.

A number of investigators in the field have suggested additional guidelines for patients to follow when choosing herbal remedies.

WHO USES HERBAL MEDICINE?

Despite the caveats regarding herbal medicine, it remains a popular choice with many who experience pain. In fact, chronic pain sufferers are more likely than those without chronic pain to use herbal treatments, as well as numerous other options from the treatment methods of complementary and alternative medicine (CAM). How do we know this?

The medical establishment is beginning to appreciate the magnitude of the use of CAM—who is using it and why. This is because medical researchers are beginning to ask patients about their use. The first mainstream medical review of this subject was published in 1993, and it brought the depth and breadth of the use of CAM therapies to the attention of the traditional American medical establishment. Many doctors were stunned to discover that about one in three patients was choosing an alternative therapy to help treat his or her medical conditions. Interestingly, almost all the patients who reported using CAM treatments also were seeking care from traditional medical doctors. Most patients that use chiropractic, massage, acupuncture, homeopathy, and other CAM treatments are also being taken care of by the medical establishment. Many surveys since 1993 have confirmed these trends. They also reveal that very few patients tell their doctors about their CAM use, and that very few doctors ask. Nonetheless, the 1993 survey showed that 34 percent of those consulting a physician for chronic pain used CAM, as did 36 percent of those with chronic back pain. A follow-up survey published in 1997 showed that rates of use were even higher.

Surveys from around the world followed and showed that the phenomenon of using alternative therapies was not limited to the United States. In fact, in some nations, use of what would be considered alternative therapies is higher than it is in the U.S., particularly when it comes to herbal therapies. This may be related to historical practices and cultural traditions. Even within the United States, the actual type of therapy chosen varies by ethnic or national group. For instance, Hispanics in the Southwest may use topical preparations of marijuana leaves soaked in alcohol for pain relief. Rural African-Americans in North Carolina may use snake venom or bee sting treatments. Midwestern city dwellers may rely on copper bracelets.

INDIVIDUAL HERBAL TREATMENTS

The following is a discussion of some individual herbal treatments that are used by patients in pain, some of which are topical and some of which may be taken orally.

Aloe Vera

Aloe vera is a common ingredient in numerous over-the-counter creams, lotions, and ointments that are intended to soothe the skin. It is a product of plants in the lily family, and commercial preparations are derived from *Aloe barbadensis.* Aloe vera has been used since ancient Greek times as a traditional treatment for wound healing, burns, and skin disorders like eczema and psoriasis. Many pharmacologically active compounds are present in aloe vera, some with anti-inflammatory properties. However, use of aloe vera may not be appropriate for all skin conditions.

More than sixty years ago, aloe vera was reported to be of benefit in a patient who had been treated with radiation and developed a significant skin rash as a result. However, more recent carefully controlled studies have not been able to demonstrate any benefit whatsoever from using aloe vera in patients receiving radiation therapy. In fact, other studies have indicated that aloe vera may be of harm in treating surgical wounds. Patients treated with aloe vera took almost 60 percent longer to heal than did patients treated with standard wound-care procedures in one study of women recovering from caesarean sections or gynecological surgery. Circumstances in which aloe vera may be of help, however, are in the healing of oral aphthous ulcers and in the healing of the initial outbreak of genital herpes. The use of topical aloe vera for widespread pain in the post-traumatic pain patient has never been studied. However, given its very modest benefits in a limited number of skin conditions, it would be unlikely to be of much overall benefit. For the present, aloe vera is best viewed as a soothing ingredient with little curative potential.

Aloe vera products for internal use also are available. These products are best avoided since there is very little scientific evidence that they are of benefit and they may cause gastrointestinal pain, diarrhea, damage to the gastrointestinal tract, and interactions with other medications.

Capsaicin

More promising as a topical adjunct for patients with diffuse pain might be products containing capsaicin. This ingredient derives from the *Capsicum* pepper family, also known as cayenne or red pepper. It is also readily available on the drugstore shelf in products claiming to reduce pain from herpes zoster, sports injuries, and arthritis, among other disorders. Capsaicin appears to have a number of pain-relieving properties. It may lead to the release of endorphins, pain-relieving substances that are naturally produced by our bodies. It also inhibits the release of substance P, a pain-producing neurotransmitter that stimulates pain nerve fibers. Patients using capsaicin-containing products experience a burning sensation at first. This sensation becomes diminished over time with repeated use, and, with several applications daily, pain can begin to subside. Repeated use is necessary, however, since the beneficial effects of capsaicin are short-lived.

Because this substance is derived from pepper plants, caution is advised when applying capsaicin to skin. It should not be applied to open wounds or broken skin. When beginning the use of capsaicin, it should be applied over a limited area of the body, for instance, over a single joint, until the user assesses its effects and side effects. Hands should be washed after use to avoid accidentally getting a capsaicin-containing product into the eyes, nose, or mouth. Finally, application of a capsaicin-containing product should not be followed by the application of heat since this can lead to an intense and unpleasant burning sensation.

Willow Bark

Many of the herbal products described in this chapter, including willow bark, are likely to derive their pain-relieving properties from the fact that they are anti-inflammatory. However, it is important to realize that there are many different ways in which a product can have an anti-inflammatory effect. Not all inflammation is alike, nor are all anti-inflammatory medicines. This is illustrated by the fact that different kinds of inflammation are present in such varying conditions as hay fever, asthma, eczema, and rheumatoid arthritis. Sometimes it is difficult to know how much of a role inflammation is playing in a particular condition, like an acutely painful herniated disc. We know that pain can certainly be present in the absence of inflammation. If this is the case, anti-inflammatory herbal treatments, no matter how effective against inflammation, are likely to be of no benefit for pain control.

Willow bark tea has been used since antiquity in the treatment of pain. Willow bark derivatives remain popular ingredients in over-the-counter arthritis preparations in the United States and Europe. This is not surprising when we consider that willow bark is a source of salicin, which is chemically related to acetylsalicylic acid, the active ingredient in aspirin. The way in which willow bark works, therefore, is thought to be similar to aspirin and the nonsteroidal anti-inflammatory drugs (NSAIDs), including the newer COX-2 inhibitors.

Research has shown that willow bark–containing preparations can be of benefit in treating the pain of osteoarthritis, the most common form of arthritis. Other work has shown that willow bark can be helpful for low back pain. We might expect, although extensive research in this area is lacking, that a painful condition that might respond to aspirin or Ibuprofen also might respond to a willow bark preparation. Conditions that have not responded to aspirinlike drugs would not be expected to do any better with willow bark treatment.

Some investigators feel that willow bark may have fewer side effects than nonsteroidal anti-inflammatory drugs. This may be because over-the-counter willow bark preparations are simply less potent than prescription NSAIDs. Getting less of the pharmacologically active ingredient might mean less of a risk of a side effect. However, a patient who has had an unacceptable side effect from over-the-counter or prescription NSAIDs should not count on willow bark to be any safer. Patients who have had a peptic ulcer, bleeding from the gastrointestinal tract, swelling of the feet, worsening of high blood pressure, or kidney problems due to NSAIDs would do well to avoid willow bark products. Patients with an allergy to aspirin should avoid preparations containing willow bark since they may be cross-reactive. In other words, they may experience the same kind of allergic reaction to willow bark.

Boron

Boron is a naturally occurring mineral present in trace amounts in human bone. It is also naturally present in fruits, vegetables, legumes, and nuts. It is used as the principal ingredient in some commercially available roach powders.

Some advocates have suggested that boron could be helpful in the treatment of pain associated with osteoarthritis. Others have suggested that it can be used to reduce the risk of osteoporosis associated with menopause. Very little information is available, however, on the exact role of boron in the body under normal circumstances, let alone what its role might be in prevention or treatment of disease.

The primary proponent of boron as an arthritis treatment is Rex E. Newham, D.O., N.D., Ph.D., who became convinced of its effectiveness after trying boron himself. He reports that it alleviated his pain, swelling, and stiffness due to arthritis and has done so for thousands of others as well. He has gathered some anecdotal evidence to support his claims, but no acceptable controlled, large-scale research has ever been done to prove a benefit. Other researchers have suggested that bones are made stronger by boron, and, therefore, that this mineral might be good for women going through menopause. However, at least one study has shown that boron supplements caused more hot flashes, more problems with sleep, including night sweats, and more overall symptoms associated with menopause.

It is also known that a boron intoxication syndrome can develop that leads to loss of motor control, drowsiness, confusion, and, in later stages, seizures. This has been described in animals and in humans given a boron overdose. It suggests that boron is best avoided until further research has been done.

Glucosamine and Chondroitin

Although glucosamine and chondroitin are not herbal products, they are among the fastest-growing and most commonly used natural products that Americans are purchasing to deal with chronic pain. They have been used in Europe for many decades and have gained in popularity since the 1997 publication of *The Arthritis Cure* by Jason Theodosakis, M.D. Glucosamine and chondroitin are not, however, useful for all types of pain. They appear to have a number of effects in the body, but their primary benefit seems to be in the treatment of pain from osteoarthritis.

Glucosamine (most commonly available as glucosamine sulfate) is a normal component of the joints and the surrounding connective tissue. In fact, glucosamine is found throughout the body. It is a normal building block of cartilage and is reduced in amount in cartilage that is affected by osteoarthritis. The glucosamine available in retail outlets is made from chitin, the hard outer shell of crustaceans. In theory, therefore, caution might be in order for those with seafood allergies who are considering using glucosamine. However, there are no reported cases of adverse reactions in seafood allergic individuals who have taken glucosamine. Similarly, some scientists have raised the theoretical concern that people with diabetes may have a loss of sugar control if they take glucosamine because it is involved in the metabolism of glucose. Again, this has not been reported in the medical literature as a significant side effect.

The way in which glucosamine works is unclear; yet many short-term studies have shown that it is effective in helping to relieve pain due to osteoarthritis. Some head-to-head comparisons with prescription medications have suggested that glucosamine works as well, but not as fast, as nonsteroidal anti-inflammatory drugs. Improvements in the level of pain, as well as in the ability to function, have been seen. Interestingly, glucosamine may have beneficial effects weeks after its usage has been stopped. Side effects in the short-term studies published so far have been minor. Usually these have included gastrointestinal upset, but no more frequently than from placebo.

One long-term study has been published, but its results remain controversial. In this three-year study conducted in Belgium, investigators found that taking glucosamine was associated with a reduced rate of arthritis progression. Those who took glucosamine had less cartilage loss on their X-rays than did those who took a placebo. Yet physicians and scientists remain unsure if cartilage is repaired or even healthier, as many health-food store labels suggest, if glucosamine is taken. Glucosamine has never been studied for its effects in counteracting other types of pain.

Nonetheless, the tremendous popularity of glucosamine has made it the supplement that health professionals themselves have asked about in my practice. One rehabilitation physician sheepishly asked me if glucosamine "worked" for arthritis. When I said it could be helpful, he admitted that he had already been using it and found it quite effective for his knee pain. Another physician colleague used it for his own chronic neck pain due to degenerative disc disease. It worked so well that he ended up using it for his arthritic dog, with considerable success.

Chondroitin (most frequently sold as chondroitin sulfate) is also a normal building block of cartilage. It too is abnormal in the cartilage of those with osteoarthritis. Again, a consumer might find it logical that replacing an abnormal component of cartilage with a supplement might be helpful. However, we know less about chondroitin than we do about glucosamine. Fewer studies have been carried out with chondroitin than glucosamine. Nonetheless, those that have been carried out similarly suggest that chondroitin can be helpful in pain relief. The benefit here, too, is comparable to that of nonsteroidal anti-inflammatory drugs, and no significant side effects have been reported. Chondroitin is made from the cartilage of cattle, and this has raised the theoretical concern that mad cow disease could be spread through its use. There has never been an instance of this occurring. Again, chondroitin has not been studied to see if it will work in pain other than the pain of arthritis. However, it does seem to be of some benefit to some individuals with osteoarthritis with a very low risk of adverse effects.

Avocado Soybean Unsaponifiables

Available in Europe, avocado soybean unsaponifiables (ASU) is popular for the treatment of osteoarthritis pain. This preparation is made from an extract of one-third avocado oil and two-thirds soybean oil; however, its actual active ingredient is unknown. This extract has been found to be a powerful anti-inflammatory drug in laboratory experiments. ASU blocks the effects of chemicals produced by the body that cause inflammation and cartilage breakdown. Rabbits given ASU were prevented from getting arthritis. Humans who have taken it in an experimental setting have had a reduction in their pain and have been able to reduce their reliance on prescription medications. Patients with knee or hip arthritis were the subjects of one study, and they significantly improved their ability to function after taking ASU for two months. ASU is available in England and France, but not in the United States. It continues to be studied by arthritis researchers.

Borage Oil and Evening Primrose Oil

In addition to the avocado soybean preparation, plant oils of other types have been investigated by researchers for their anti-inflammatory properties. A number of plants are sources of a particular type of fatty acid that can be converted by the body into anti-inflammatory agents. This omega-6 fatty acid is called gamma linolenic acid (GLA) and is present in borage seed oil, evening primrose oil, and black currant seed oil. Borage oil has the highest concentration of this substance. Use of these oils in folk medicine included both topical and oral use. There is no scientific evidence, however, that rubbing the body or the joints with these oils makes any difference in pain. However, reports on a number of well-performed clinical research studies document that at least evening primrose oil and borage oil can reduce pain and swelling in patients with rheumatoid arthritis (RA). Patients with inflammatory arthritis also have been able to reduce their need for prescription medications by using these oils. We do not know if these plant oils are helpful if taken internally for any other types of pain.

Side effects have included an increased risk of bleeding. These oils thin the blood. This by itself may put a user at risk for bleeding. This is an even more important risk in patients on other drugs that have an effect on blood clotting. These drugs include warfarin (Coumadin), heparin, low molecular weight heparin (Lovenox), aspirin, nonsteroidal anti-inflammatory drugs, and herbal medicines that have effects on blood (garlic, ginger, and turmeric).

Fish Oil

Plants are not the only source of anti-inflammatory oils. Fish—in particular, those from deep ocean waters—contain anti-inflammatory oils as well. Many scientific studies have shown that fish oil can reduce pain and inflammation in patients with rheumatoid arthritis. How well fish oil works for other types of arthritis or other types of pain has not been studied, however. Fish oils contain omega-3 fatty acids, including eicosapentaenoic acid (EPA) and docosahexaenoic acid (DHA). Flaxseed contains a fatty acid that is a building block of EPA, but it has not been studied to the extent that fish oils have. These fatty acids are a normal part of the cell wall in the body. They can be used by cells to make anti-inflammatory substances. As with the plant oils mentioned above, research shows that taking fish oil can reduce pain and inflammation in people with rheumatoid arthritis. RA patients have also been able to reduce their reliance on prescription nonsteroidal anti-inflammatory drugs when taking fish oil.

Large doses of fish oil are required to get noticeable anti-inflammatory benefits. The doses needed often lead to unacceptable gastrointestinal side effects. Furthermore, the same caution must be used when choosing fish oil as an anti-inflammatory as pertains to plant oils: Blood thinning may occur. This is an important potential side effect in the absence of any other disease or medication. It should be considered even more seriously when patients are on other medications that can thin the blood or have had significant medical conditions that led to bleeding. Medications that could interact with fish oil include warfarin (Coumadin), heparin, low molecular weight heparin (Lovenox), aspirin, nonsteroidal anti-inflammatory drugs, and herbal medicines that have effects on blood (garlic, ginger, and turmeric). An important medical condition to consider in this regard is any history of previous bleeding, including a hemorrhagic stroke or peptic ulcer. Anyone thinking about taking plant or animal oils that can affect bleeding should discuss their use with their physician beforehand.

HELPFUL WEB SITES

ConsumerLab.com

http://www.consumerlab.com

ConsumerLab.com states that its mission is to identify the best-quality health and nutrition products through independent testing. This site publishes results of its tests for labeling accuracy, purity, bioavailability, and consistency online, including listing of brands that have passed testing. Products tested include herbal preparations, vitamins, minerals, other supplements, sports and energy products, other foods and beverages, and personal-care products.

Dr. Theo Online

http://www.drtheo.com

This Web site is maintained by Dr. Jason Theodosakis who introduced the idea of using glucosamine and chondroitin for treatment of arthritis pain to the American public with his book The Arthritis Cure. *He has independently tested several brands of these products and has published his results on this site. In addition, general information about glucosamine and chondroitin and arthritis treatment is available here.*

Food and Drug Administration MedWatch

http://www.fda.gov/medwatch

MedWatch is a site of the U.S. Food and Drug Administration Medical Products Reporting Program. This program was established to disseminate information to health professionals and consumers about safety issues involving medical products, including prescription and over-the-counter drugs, biologics, dietary supplements, and medical devices. Safety information dating to reports from 1996 on recalls, withdrawals, and labeling changes is available. Consumers and health professionals also may report serious problems suspected to be related to medications or devices.

Tufts University Health & Nutrition Letter

http://www.healthletter.tufts.edu

This monthly newsletter gives consumers the latest, scientifically based information on health and disease, nutrition, and supplements and products related to these fields. This newsletter is available by subscription. Subscribers may submit their health and nutrition questions to the editors.

15

Ayurvedic Medicine

ARVIND CHOPRA, M.D.
(WITH JAYSHREE PATIL, M.D.)

The term Ayurveda in the ancient Indian language of Sanskrit means knowledge *(veda)* of life *(ayur)*. During the prebiblical ancient Hindu civilization era, the Ayurvedic texts were written in Sanskrit (considered to be the mother of all languages used in India today). Centuries later, these texts exist, but probably much has been lost or transformed. Much of the current Ayurveda text is considered to have originated during the period 1000–6000 B.C. However, Ayurveda is a thriving and popular medicinal system in India. Ayurveda has its own network of medical colleges and hospitals with well-established curriculum for both graduate and postgraduate study.

Ayurveda is a holistic science that promotes health through appropriate diet and lifestyle. Exercise and personal hygiene are emphasized. Mental discipline and control and adherence to moral and spiritual values are prerequisites for good health. Ayurveda also promotes the practices of rejuvenation (rasayana) and virilification (vajikarana) in daily life. The understanding of "prakriti" of every individual is critical to both health and disease. While prakriti signifies "constitution," it also means "nature" and conceptually unifies all matter.

The "tridosha" theory (*tri* means three, and *dosha* is equivalent to a biological humor) is the core concept in health and disease. The three "doshas"—that is, "vata," "pitta," and "kapha"—are considered to govern the bio-motor, the metabolic and the preservative (homeostasis) activity respectively as the primary physiological forces. Each dosha has its own characteristic anatomical, physiological, and psychological expressions. The "prakriti" of each individual is driven by the dominant dosha, and any imbalance in the three doshas causes disease.

The "tridosha" theory is fundamental to the understanding of disease in Ayurveda. The Ayurvedic treatment is highly individualized because the ancients believed that no two individuals suffered from apparently similar disease. Thus, great emphasis has been placed on the diagnosis *(nidan)*, which is based on detailed history, on clinical examination, and, most important, on the conclusions regarding the deranged dosha and prakriti of the individual. Deviations in diet and behavior pattern from Ayurvedic norms also are evaluated for targeting therapy.

BASIC THERAPY

Some of the orthodox therapies in practice today remain quite unchanged from the ancient treatments; besides being complex and time consuming, they are difficult to standardize and cumbersome to administer.

Treatment usually begins with the two basic processes—"svedna" (sweating and heating) and "snehana" (lubrication). While diaphoretic, steam bath, and so on may be used to execute the former, oily preparations are administered orally and/or through medicated enemas and massages to execute the latter. These processes aim at cleansing and purifying the body. The drugs are administered to patients through multiple routes concurrently or sequentially. Extracts of medicinal plants are often added to the drug vehicle (often oils, butter, curds, and milk) and administered as enemas. Guided by the therapeutic response, the various procedures described above are often repeated cyclically.

Dietary restrictions form the mainstay of treatment, and physical exercises and yoga are advocated to promote recovery and healing. Some patients with acute painful rheumatic-musculoskeletal (RMS) conditions or inflammatory arthritis are often required to fast *(langhana)* in the initial stage to strengthen the digestive and metabolic systems. Similarly, some patients are offered a special, easily digestible diet.

Pain is considered a multifaceted dimension, and its relief is given prime importance. The neuropsychological factors have been described in the ancient literature, and some fascinating healing methods have been advocated: For example, "the patient lying on a bed moistened with dews of moonrays covered with flax and lotus leaves and fanned with breeze cooled by contact of sandy beach should be attended by beloved and sweet spoken women with their breasts and hands pasted with sandal and with cold and pleasing touch who remove burning sensation, pain and exhaustion." We are not aware of such techniques currently being practiced anywhere in India, but they do prompt us to emphasize the non-pharmacological means of reducing pain that appear to have been forgotten by modern medicine.

Some of the medicinal plant extracts used to relieve pain and inflammation in Ayurvedic medicine are listed in Table 15.1. Local applications to painful regions of the body are very popular, and poultices enclosed in leaves of some of these medicinal plants are liberally applied. The latter is also an important component of the various tribal systems of medicine practiced in India today.

Substandard commercial Ayurvedic formulations are often sold as over-the-counter drugs and sometimes test positive for surreptitiously mixed steroids and NSAIDs. Ayurvedic doctors often coprescribe modern medicines for quick response.

THE ANCIENT AYURVEDA did deal with the pain and swelling components of trauma and many other medical disorders. In the current context, it seems that the analgesic attributes of some of the Ayurvedic formulations in use today, as compared with those of modern-day analgesics, are modest but extremely safe in the long run. The anti-inflammatory properties of Ayurvedic mineral/plant–based formulations are more impressive.

Recent publications have tried to convey the relevance of the science of Ayurvedic herbalism to the needs of modern times. The ancient com-

TABLE 15.1 SINGLE PLANT EXTRACTS USED TO RELIEVE PAIN AND INFLAMMATION

No.	Plant	Dominant Effect
1	Ajmoda (*Carum roxburghianum*)	Analgesic
2	Arka (*Calotropis procera*)	Analgesic, Anti-inflammatory
3	Aragvadha (*Cassia fistula*)	Analgesic, Anti-inflammatory
4	Karpoor (*Cinamomum camphora*)	Analgesic
5	Jyotishmati (*Celastrus paniculata*)	Analgesic
6	Nimba (*Azadirachta indica*)	Anti-inflammatory
7	Lavang (*Syzygium aromaticum*)	Analgesic
8	Vacha (*Acorus calamus*)	Analgesic, Anti-inflammatory
9	Shigru (*Moringa oleifera*)	Analgesic, Anti-inflammatory
10	Peelu (*Salvadora persica*)	Analgesic, Anti-inflammatory

plex Ayurvedic treatments would necessarily have to be clinically validated before they could fulfill the needs of modern humans. However, a futuristic medical system of modern medicine–Ayurveda medicine has already begun to emerge, at least in the Eastern part of the world.

SUGGESTED READINGS

Chopra, A. "Ayurvedic Medicine and Arthritis," *Rheumatic Diseases Clinics of North America* 2000; 26(1):133–144.

Gogte, V.M. *Ayurvedic Pharmacology and Therapeutic Uses of Medicinal Plants* (English translation). Mumbai, India: Bharatiya Vidya Bhawan, 2000.

Lele, R.D. "Ayurveda Through Modern Eyes," in *Ayurveda and Modern Medicine.* Bombay: Bharatiya Vidya Bhawan, 1986.

Sharma, S. *The System of Ayurveda.* Delhi, India: Low Price Publications, 1995.

16

Chiropractic Care

BRUCE PFLEGER, PH.D.

The idea of restoring health by delivering a forceful thrust to an area of the spine is centuries old, dating at least to ancient Greece. In 400 B.C., Hippocrates recommended that patients with a hump in their backs lie on a wooden bed while a strong, skilled physician or an assistant delivers pressure to the raised area to reduce it. Hippocrates's descriptions of hand positioning and the direction of the thrust are remarkably similar to procedures that chiropractors use today.

The birth date of the chiropractic profession is considered to be September 18, 1895, when Daniel David ("D.D.") Palmer was treating a patient who was complaining of hearing loss. Palmer reported that when he delivered a thrust to a bump on the patient's neck, the patient's hearing was restored. Inspired by this result, Palmer coined the term "chiropractic" with the help of a minister, combining the Greek words *chiros* (hands) and *praktikos* (pertaining to action). Thus, chiropractic, a word that can be used as a noun or adjective, means "done by hand." Palmer founded several chiropractic schools, including the Palmer School of Chiropractic, which still exists today in Davenport, Iowa.

Chiropractic is now the third-largest health profession in the United

States, after medicine and dentistry. Unlike medicine and dentistry, the chiropractic profession remains free of drugs and surgery. About 60,000 professionals who hold the degree of Doctor of Chiropractic (D.C.) practice in the United States, in addition to many others throughout the world.

LOCATING THE CAUSE OF PAIN

At first, a visit with a chiropractor might seem a little confusing: For example, if your arm hurts, you might wonder why a chiropractor would work on your neck. Or you might ask, "What does my back have to do with the burning in my legs?" Chiropractors use a wide assortment of techniques and therapies; however, their practice is rooted in the belief that a properly functioning spine and nervous system will allow your body to heal itself of most problems.

A patient who consults both a chiropractor and a medical doctor for the same injuries will receive two different courses of treatment. For example, Gary was injured in a car accident. Athough he was wearing his seat belt, he suffered bumps and bruises when his body hit the steering wheel. The muscles in his back and neck feel stiff, and he has frequent headaches. When Gary sees a medical doctor, he will provide information about previous injuries and illnesses and will receive a physical examination. He also might undergo X-rays or provide blood and urine for laboratory analysis. Each of these tests will assist his medical doctor in diagnosing Gary's injuries.

Physicians use diagnoses to provide a systematic means of describing injuries or diseases, which they then treat. Along with the diagnosis—such as a contusion (bruise) of the thorax (chest)—the doctor records associated symptoms such as pain, tenderness, and swelling. Assuming that Gary has no broken bones or other serious injuries, he might receive a medication such as an analgesic to reduce head and body pain, a muscle relaxant to help with stiffness, and anti-inflammatory pills to help reduce swelling.

Contrast this approach with Gary's experience when he visits a chiropractor. The doctor of chiropractic will take a history and perform a physical examination similar to that of a medical doctor but will pay more attention to the bones, muscles, and other tissues near Gary's spine. In all likelihood, the chiropractor will not list the same diagnoses that a medical doctor would. In fact, many states restrict chiropractors from making such diagnoses because they lack the in-depth training necessary to do so. Instead, the chiropractor will look primarily for misalignments of bones in Gary's joints. If misalignments are found, the chiropractor will try to realign the joints. For example, a rib might be out of place, producing pain, or a bone in the back might be twisted, resulting in spastic muscles.

The philosophy of chiropractic is based on the concept that joint misalignments can result in pain, discomfort, nerve interference, and even diseases, and that realignment of the joints can eliminate the symptoms of these disorders. While a medical doctor probably will prescribe pills to help Gary reduce symptoms of pain, swelling, and stiffness, a chiropractor will seek to remove the *cause* of the symptoms. This is why chiropractors say that they don't "treat" diseases but instead seek to alleviate the underlying source of the problem.

Many chiropractors also provide preventive care in the belief that putting a person's spine and other joints in perfect alignment will mean fewer health problems in the future. Just as good oral hygiene can prevent tooth decay, many chiropractors believe that good posture and regular examinations by a chiropractor could help maintain health. However, the role of chiropractic in prevention is not well accepted outside the profession, or even within it.

Most chiropractors would agree that their primary role is to detect and to subsequently correct or reduce partial dislocations of the spine. The Association of Chiropractic Colleges, representing all seventeen chiropractic schools in North America, defines chiropractic practice thusly: "The practice of chiropractic focuses on the relationship between structure (primarily of the spine) and function (as coordinated by the nervous system) and how that relationship affects the preservation and restoration of health."

The relative position of joints is essential to this relationship. An anatomical joint is the place where two or more bones come together, separated by tissue such as cartilage or by liquid called synovial fluid. When the bones of a joint are moved sufficiently so that their surfaces are no longer in contact, a dislocation, or luxation, occurs. More than three hundred years ago, medical literature began to refer to a partial dislocation, one in which bones are displaced but still in contact, as a subluxation.

Today, the term "vertebral subluxation complex" is often used to describe not only joint displacement but also associated changes in the adjoining muscles, blood vessels, nerves, and connective tissues. However, the term "subluxation" often is used simply to refer to a dislocation that a chiropractor seeks to correct.

LICENSING AND ACCREDITATION

Chiropractic is licensed in all fifty states and in many foreign countries. In the United States, chiropractors act as independent providers, meaning that they do not require supervision by another health-care provider.

Chiropractors must hold a valid license from the state in which they practice. To become a licensed practitioner, a chiropractor must graduate from an accredited program. The United States currently has sixteen programs for chiropractic studies that are accredited by the Counsel on Chiropractic Education (CCE), an agency recognized by the U.S. Department of Education. The CCE sets standards for coursework, faculty and staff, facilities, patient care, and research.

Graduates of chiropractor programs receive a Doctor of Chiropractic (D.C.) degree. Some parts of the chiropractic curriculum are similar to those required for a Doctor of Medicine (M.D.) degree, but chiropractors receive more hours of training in anatomy, and no training in pharmacology. Chiropractic students are required to complete 4,200 hours of instruction in anatomy; biochemistry; physiology; microbiology; pathology; public health; physical, clinical, and laboratory diagnosis; gynecology; obstetrics; pediatrics; geriatrics; dermatology; otolaryngology; diagnostic imaging procedures, including radiology; psychology; nutrition/dietetics; biomechanics; orthopedics; neurology; first-aid and emergency procedures; spinal analysis; principles and practice of chiropractic; clinical decision-making; adjustive techniques; research methods and procedures; and professional ethics.

Graduates of chiropractor programs must pass national board examinations and, in some states, state board exams. Each state's chiropractic governing body controls the types of procedures that chiropractors may use within that state; for example, some states are very restrictive, while others allow chiropractors to use a wider variety of procedures, including acupuncture.

EXAMINATION BY A CHIROPRACTOR

Because chiropractors act as primary-care providers, patients can see them without a referral from a medical doctor or other health-care professional. However, it is common for medical doctors, massage therapists, and others to refer their patients to chiropractors, especially for relief of back and neck pain. Chiropractors can be located through the yellow pages and other advertising media, through state and national organizations, and through Internet-based finder programs like the ones listed under "Helpful Web Sites and Organizations" on page 248. An appointment usually is necessary, although some chiropractors will see patients on a "walk-in" basis.

During your first visit, a chiropractor will begin by asking a series of questions about the aspects of health that are of greatest concern to you, as well as questions about your history of health and injuries, your family medical history, your diet and exercise habits, your sleeping habits, your job, and stresses in your life. This will be followed by a physical examination, with close attention to your back and neck.

A chiropractor is primarily interested in the relative positioning of the bones that provide support to the body, including the bones of the skull; the bones of the pelvis (hips); and the twenty-seven vertebrae that make up the spinal column: three sacral (tail), five lumbar (low back), twelve thoracic (mid-upper back), and seven cervical (neck).

Chiropractors use many methods to detect abnormal alignment and movement patterns in the spine. Most commonly, D.C.s use their hands to palpate (touch) the tissues surrounding the spine. They look for areas that are tender, swollen, or inflamed. They examine vertebrae to see if they are misaligned or if their movement is hindered or abnormal. Additionally, many chiropractors assess range of motion, postural symmetry, and deficiencies in walking motion. While the patient is lying down, the D.C. also looks to see if one leg appears longer than the other, which could indicate that the muscles on one side of the body are twisting the pelvis.

Chiropractors also may use a variety of other techniques or studies in determining a diagnosis. Most common are X-ray studies, which are frequently made for new patients as well as for existing patients who have developed a new condition. Radiology is a significant part of chiropractic education, and some chiropractic adjusting techniques rely upon X-ray analysis to identify misalignment. X-rays also can identify conditions in which chiropractic adjustment in a certain area may be dangerous, such as severe osteoporosis or spinal tumor. Other imaging techniques, such as CT (computerized tomography) scans or MRI (magnetic resonance imaging), are used less frequently. Many chiropractors also use laboratory values derived from blood and urine screenings, especially to rule out life-threatening conditions. However, many states preclude chiropractors from performing invasive tests such as drawing blood.

DIAGNOSIS

The primary diagnosis that chiropractors draw from their examinations is subluxation in the spinal column. This diagnosis is largely independent of the reasons that patients give for seeking treatment and the symptoms they describe. Other commonly made diagnoses include strains and sprains, tendinitis, problems with intervertebral discs that provide cushions between the bony vertebrae, joint degeneration, and other conditions that relate primarily to the spinal column.

Chiropractors have a broad education and can diagnose common diseases and conditions. However, they lack the knowledge and equipment necessary to diagnose rare or complicated conditions, and many states prohibit chiropractors from making diagnoses. If a chiropractor thinks that a disease or condition is present that requires care from another health-care professional, either within the chiropractic profession or from another profession, the D.C. will refer the patient to an appropriate health-care provider. However, chiropractors are generally willing to provide care for those with a variety of diseases, as long as there is evidence of the need for spinal adjustments. Even if a referral is made, a D.C. usually will offer a patient chiropractic care. For instance, upon examining a patient, a chiropractor might suspect a blood disorder, which requires a specialist in the medical profession. Yet the D.C. would still want to correct any spinal misalignments that could be interfering with the body's ability to function at its maximal level.

ADJUSTMENT TECHNIQUES

Health-care professionals use several terms to describe various therapies for the spine. "Mobilization" is a technique of moving a joint within its normal range of motion and is practiced most often by physiotherapists, massage therapists, and osteopaths. For example, if a spinal joint is fixated or "stuck" so that no movement can take place, a physical therapist using mobilization therapy will apply force to the joint until the fixation "breaks" and the joint is free to move again through normal twisting and bending motions.

"Manipulation" generally refers to applying force to take a joint past its normal range of motion. This method, used by all professionals who apply manual pressure to the spine and other joints, often results in a popping sound like the sound you hear when you "crack" your knuckles. The term "spinal manipulative therapy" is a general term describing manual methods to move vertebrae.

Most chiropractors prefer the term "adjustment," which implies an alignment procedure designed to restore the functions of the skeletal and nervous systems. Chiropractors often make an analogy to the workings of fine machinery: Manipulating the controls can change the functioning of a machine, albeit in a fairly random manner, whereas adjusting the controls can make the machine work more efficiently.

The chiropractic profession recognizes at least a hundred adjustment techniques, many of which are named for the pioneers who developed systems for assessing each type of misalignment as well as procedures to correct the misalignments. Most of these techniques are designed to correct spinal misalignments, but the same principles can be applied to other joints, especially in the arms and legs.

It's worth noting that the sensation of pain occurs in the brain. Each pain receptor in the skin, muscles, and organs is connected to the spinal cord by a neuron, which connects to a second neuron that travels to the brain. When you feel pain from a certain location, it could be that the pain receptor is being stimulated, or it could be that either of the two neurons connecting the receptor to your brain is being stimulated. In other words, a pain that you feel in your foot might be caused by something pressing on your spinal cord. For this reason, a chiropractic adjustment at a certain level of your spinal cord could affect pain sensation (and muscle and other tissue functions) for all the nerves that enter the spinal cord *below* the level being adjusted. So a pain or a muscle spasm in your foot could be caused by an injury to your neck.

All chiropractors use adjusting techniques, but individual practitioners use these techniques in three different ways. In the first of these, the D.C.

CATEGORIES OF ADJUSTING TECHNIQUES

1. Full-spine techniques, to adjust vertebrae in the spine at the point where nerves from the area of pain enter the spinal cord.
2. Full-spine techniques, using information from X-rays, to adjust vertebrae in the spine that are out of alignment with adjoining vertebrae.
3. Techniques to adjust one primary area of the spine, such as the uppermost vertebrae, to realign the entire spine.

identifies the location on the patient's body that is in pain or distress and adjusts the area of the spine from which nerves exit the spinal cord and travel to the affected area. For instance, after slipping and falling on the ice, a person might complain of sharp, persistent pain in the buttocks. A chiropractor, knowing that the nerve cells that sense pain in the buttocks enter the spinal cord at the level of the top vertebra in the lower back, would apply chiropractic adjustments to that spinal segment in an effort to relieve the pressure on the nerve root exiting the spinal cord.

The second category of adjusting techniques concerns those based on diagnosis of specific misalignments that have been identified in the spinal column. Based primarily on analysis of X-rays but also on examination by touch and analysis of posture, D.C.s adjust those vertebrae that appear out of alignment with respect to the vertebrae located directly above and below. The goal is to align the spine as straight as possible, with the expectation that pain and/or other symptoms will then disappear.

It's not unusual for a chiropractor to provide identical care to two patients who have greatly differing reasons for seeking help. One person might complain of constant fatigue, while another complains of stomach problems. However, upon examination, the chiropractor might find that in both cases the sixth cervical vertebra (a neck bone) is twisted and pushed to the side. The chiropractor would then try to realign that vertebra, and either or both patients might benefit.

The first two categories of adjustment techniques incorporate so-called "full-spine" techniques, in which a chiropractor might adjust one or more vertebrae in the spine. Chiropractors who use the third category of adjusting techniques favor adjusting at one specific site, regardless of

A CASE IN POINT: A PAIN IN THE BACK

After suffering minor injuries in an automobile accident, Elena visits a chiropractor because of pain in her lower back.

The D.C. she consults is an upper-cervical specialist who primarily adjusts only the top two bones in the neck. In looking at Elena's standing posture and X-rays of her spine, the D.C. sees that Elena has two lateral curves, one in her neck and a second in her lower back. The one in her neck, the primary curvature, is caused by the skull being misaligned with the top cervical vertebra. This has the effect of tilting her head to the right. But Elena lives in the modern world, driving, reading, and watching television, all of which are hard to do with your head tilted to one side. So, without realizing it, she has been trying to compensate by leaning to the left, and a secondary curvature has developed in her lower back in the opposite direction, putting her eyes at their original level. The secondary curve in her lower back is responsible for her pain.

The D.C. is successful in realigning Elena's skull with the top cervical vertebra. This has the temporary effect of tilting Elena's head to the left, because of the still-existing secondary curvature. However, within a week or so, the curve in her back disappears on its own, and with it goes the pain.

In this example, the patient consulted an upper-cervical specialist. However, some chiropractors adjust primarily the pelvis, or the base of the spine, with the idea that if the base of the spine is straight, the rest of the spine will straighten out as well.

the reason that the patient came in for treatment. The philosophy of this technique is that if the bones in this primary site are aligned, the rest of the spine will respond and align itself accordingly.

Within the three categories of adjusting techniques, many individual chiropractic techniques are used, varying in their methods of analysis and the way that force is delivered to the joint. Most techniques involve positioning the hands to apply force directly to the vertebra, using the spinous processes—the little pieces of bone sticking out of the vertebrae—as levers to generate movement and rotation. The force may be applied quickly or slowly. Additionally, a D.C. might use a customized table equipped with movable segments that lift or drop while the adjustment is being made to assist with the desired movement. Other techniques include using a handheld or table-mounted instrument to deliver the force. Last, some techniques apply massagelike pressures to muscles connected to the vertebra, causing relaxation and indirectly promoting movement of the bones.

In addition to making spinal adjustments, chiropractors use other methods of care. Ice packs are frequently used. Other forms of treatment that are used by more than half the profession, in descending frequency of usage, are trigger-point therapy (a form of massage for muscles and nerves), nutritional counseling, bracing (back or neck support), massage therapy, hot packs, traction, electrical stimulation, bed rest, heel lifts, mobilization therapy, ultrasound, acupressure or meridian therapy, and homeopathic remedies.

A PLAN OF CARE

Most conditions will require multiple trips to a chiropractor. The first visit is usually the longest, because that is when a chiropractor takes a patient's history and performs a physical examination. These are extremely important in identifying conditions that need urgent attention.

After reviewing the patient's medical history and analyzing X-rays and any other imaging and laboratory information, a chiropractor makes an initial diagnosis and will form a care plan for a number of visits to be scheduled over subsequent days and weeks.

In most cases, the first adjustment is made on the first day. Adjustments are usually done with the patient positioned on a table specifically designed to assist certain chiropractic techniques. The patient may be asked to lie on his or her stomach, back, or side; some techniques use a table that the patient leans against in a kneeling position. Precise positioning is very important, as it helps to open the joint being adjusted, reducing the amount of force needed for the adjustment. The D.C. might stretch or massage a joint to further enable joint movement. The adjusting procedure is done by producing a force, either with the hands or with an instrument. This may be repeated until the D.C. senses that the desired vertebral motion has been made.

Usually adjustment is not painful, although it may cause some discomfort. Chiropractic education stresses warm doctor-patient relations, and patients often enjoy their sessions with chiropractors. Various studies have shown that patients are more satisfied with their chiropractors than with their medical doctors, probably because chiropractors generally spend more time with their patients and have more physical contact with them.

After performing an adjustment, many chiropractors ask the patient to remain on the table or to move to another comfortable location for a rest period. Based on the success of the initial care, the D.C. schedules additional visits. Advice about exercise, diet, sleeping position, ergonomics, and activities to avoid is also given at this time.

There is no way of knowing how many visits will be needed to correct a certain condition. It will depend upon many factors, including the severity of the condition, the chiropractic technique used, and the individual response of the patient. Usually, the D.C. is most interested in seeing patients "hold an adjustment." D.C.s try to correct spinal misalignments, and for some time after an adjustment, the spine has a tendency to revert to its misaligned state. Some D.C.s believe that a single adjustment is sufficient for most of their patients; others prefer that patients return periodically for the rest of their lives. Usually, the frequency of visits will be high initially, perhaps two or three visits a week for a few weeks, then tapering off to perhaps once a month, with visits discontinuing when the chiropractor and patient agree that maximal improvement has occurred.

The care phase has three stages: acute, reconstructive, and preventive/maintenance. In the acute phase, patients with post-traumatic pain experience tenderness, inflammation, and restrictions in their normal activities because of pain and swelling. During this phase, the D.C. uses therapies designed to help reduce pain and inflammation, such as cold packs, and it could be impractical to use certain adjusting techniques at this stage.

During the reconstructive phase, a chiropractor focuses on adjusting the spine to eliminate misalignments. As patients begin to "hold" their adjustments for longer periods of time, the frequency of visits decreases.

The maintenance phase occurs after a patient has achieved maximal improvement and is offered to help optimize health by correcting misalignments before symptoms appear. A good chiropractor evaluates the care plan at each visit and checks to see if the patient is making adequate progress. If progress is not being made, the care plan should be altered or the patient should be referred to another health-care professional.

PAYING FOR CHIROPRACTIC CARE

Most insurance plans provide some coverage for chiropractic services. In addition, chiropractic is covered by the federal programs Medicaid, Medicare, and Workers' Compensation. Federal civil-service employees are granted sick leave based on chiropractic certification, and chiropractic care can be included as a medical cost in calculating federal income-tax deductions.

Two studies have shown that 21 to 28 percent of payments to chiropractors are paid by patients, with the balance paid by private health insurance, auto insurance, federal health-care programs such as Workers' Compensation, managed-care insurance, and other sources.

BENEFITS AND SAFETY

The scientific community has concluded that chiropractic care is beneficial in a number of situations. Based on research studies, the Agency for Healthcare Research and Quality (AHRQ), a part of the U.S. Department of Health and Human Services, found that for uncomplicated, acute back pain of less than three months' duration, patients preferred chiropractic care to medical treatment. Evidence demonstrates that chiropractic care results in a higher probability of recovery, and that the benefits last longer, than relief offered in the form of medication. For those who have chronic back pain—longer than three months' duration—chiropractic helps reduce pain, but its long-term effects are not clear.

For relief of neck pain, studies have shown that manipulation can decrease the sensation of pain and increase neck mobility. Headache research also has shown chiropractic to be beneficial: In one study, patients who received chiropractic care experienced more relief from headaches than those who received the medication amitriptyline. Moreover, the chiropractic group experienced long-lasting relief, whereas the effects of the medicine wore off once patients stopped taking it. Whether a headache arises in the neck or is of the migraine type, chiropractic appears beneficial.

Patients with whiplash injury also are good candidates for chiropractic care. Whiplash is a common result of trauma, especially automobile accidents, but this injury is difficult to diagnose because damage to tissues often does not show up on X-rays. Although many people recover from whiplash without treatment, others experience pain and restricted mobility for months or even years. Immobilization with neck collars is not recommended, as this causes adhesions to develop in the tissues, which could permanently restrict motion. Instead, evidence indicates that mobilization and manipulation help increase range of motion, with manipulation resulting in greater reduction of pain.

Although the chiropractic profession lacks a systemic means to account for serious complications following care, rough estimates based on the number of serious events reported compared with the number of adjustments performed indicate that chiropractic care is safe, especially compared with treatments involving medication or surgery.

The most common serious event is compromise of the vertebrobasilar artery, which results in stroke or death about once in every one million adjustments. Some evidence suggests that adjustments by rotation of the skull may be responsible for most of these cases.

Complications following adjustments in the neck have occurred, but are rare. Even more rare is cauda equina syndrome, which involves the spinal nerves at the base of the spine and which occurs at a rate of about once in 100 million low-back adjustments. Typically, surgical decompression reduces symptoms of cauda equina syndrome but leaves patients with mild constipation or partial paralysis.

Imaging studies such as X-rays and CT scans impose a small but recognized risk for cancer. Currently, no strong evidence shows that chiropractic care based on X-ray analysis is superior to care that does not use X-rays. Still, it should be recognized that X-ray analysis is essential to many of the techniques used in the chiropractic profession, and excluding X-rays from a care plan before more research can be done on their comparative effectiveness is probably premature.

One further safety issue is the inability of chiropractors to detect serious conditions that require urgent medical attention. Patients who experience injuries resulting from severe trauma are advised to seek medical care prior to or in addition to chiropractic care. Of course, you also should seek medical attention if you suspect that you have a life-threatening disease.

Chiropractic is associated with few harmful side effects and has been shown to be beneficial in treating certain injuries. If it results in reduced use of medications that are associated with harmful side effects, its usefulness is clearly enhanced.

SUGGESTED READINGS

Bigos, S., Bowyer, O., Braen, G., et al. *Acute Low Back Problems in Adults. Clinical Practice Guideline No. 14.* AHCPR publication no. 95-0642. Rockville, MD: Agency for Health Care Policy and Research, Public Health Service, U.S. Department of Health and Human Services, December 1994.

Chiropractic in the United States: Training, Practice, and Research. Research Summary. Rockville, MD: Agency for Health Care Policy and Research. Information and ordering: http://www.ahrq.gov/clinic/chiropr.htm. Internet link to document: www.chiroweb.com/archives/ahcpr/uschiros.htm.

Kaptchuk, Ted J., Eisenberg, David M. "Chiropractic: Origins, Controversies, and Contributions," *Archives of Internal Medicine* 1998; 158 (20):2215–24.

Lawrence, Dana. "Chiropractic Medicine," in Jonas, Wayne B., and Levin, Jeffrey S., eds. *Essentials of Complementary and Alternative Medicine.* Philadelphia, PA: Lippincott Williams and Wilkins, 1999.

Redwood, Daniel, ed. *Contemporary Chiropractic.* New York: Churchill Livingstone, 1997.

HELPFUL WEB SITES AND ORGANIZATIONS

American Chiropractic Association
1701 Clarendon Blvd.
Arlington, VA 22209
Telephone: 800-986-4636
Fax: 703-243-2593
http://www.amerchiro.org

Association of Chiropractic Colleges
http://www.chirocolleges.org

ChiroACCESS
http://www.chiroaccess.com

Links and search of chiropractic literature.

Chiropractor Locator
http://www.chiroweb.com/locator/index.php

Council on Chiropractic Education
8049 North 85th Way
Scottsdale, AZ 85258-4321
Telephone: 480-443-8877
Fax: 480-483-7333
E-mail: cce@cce-usa.org
http://www.cce-usa.org

Web site contains links to all accredited chiropractic institutions along with their current accreditation status.

Foundation for Chiropractic Education and Research
704 E. 4th Street
Des Moines, IA 50309
E-mail: FCERNow@aol.com
http://www.fcer.org

International Chiropractors Association
1110 North Glebe Rd., Suite 1000
Arlington, VA 22201
Telephone: 800-423-4690 or 703-528-5000
Fax: 703-528-5023
http://www.chiropractic.com

National Board of Chiropractic Examiners
901 54th Avenue
Greeley, CO 80634
Telephone: 970-356-9100
http://www.nbce.org

National Center for Complementary and Alternative Medicine
http://nccam.nih.gov

Part of the National Institutes of Health.

World Chiropractic Alliance
2950 N. Dobson Rd., Suite 1
Chandler, AZ 85224
Telephone: 800-347-1011
Fax: 480-732-9313
http://www.worldchiropracticalliance.org

17

Yoga

MARIAN GARFINKEL, ED.D.

You may think of a yoga practitioner as someone sitting in a lotus position with legs tied in knots, or someone in a headstand position. Yoga, however, is more than performing strange contortions, walking on hot coals, or living in caves. Yoga is an ancient and traditional practice that is for everyone who needs energy, strength, and clarity of mind.

Yoga therapy has led to improvement in various conditions and body functioning such as raising the threshold of pain and endurance. It can be useful in treating post-traumatic pain. It calms the brain and soothes the nerves, reducing the anticipation of pain. It allows the human system to function more efficiently. This method of therapy takes more time, but the results can be longer lasting. The aim is not only to cure the specific system but also to treat the cause. The beauty of a method like yoga is that an action that focuses on one layer of our system may influence another layer in a positive way.

Yoga is an efficient technique for releasing tension from the body and creating a calm mind. It is a system for total development—physically, mentally, and spiritually—for anyone who wants a more balanced and harmonious life. It is ideal for exploring one's self: to get to know how one's body and mind respond to various experiences. Learning mastery of the body and taking control of the mind give one independence through life's various challengers. "Yoga is the golden key which unlocks the door to peace, tranquility and joy," according to BKS Iyengar.

Coping pressures and demands of daily living often create mental and physical pain and stress. This stress makes itself felt in our bodies. Weakness, stiffness, and loss of mobility and strength can be depressing. If the flow of energy is interrupted, we become tense. The ancient system of yoga techniques can help promote strength, stamina, flexibility, and emotional fortitude.

Yoga can complement any form of exercise, physical sport, or various kinds of therapy. Through a sequence of yoga postures *(asanas)*, the physical body is stretched with awareness of alignment, precision, and balance. Muscles are lengthened, circulation is improved, and energy is increased. Regular practice of yoga asanas improves concentration, benefiting both body and mind. As one practices more deeply, lightness can be felt in the body. One may develop a healthier way of eating, thinking, and acting. It is possible to change one's behavior, attitude, and general approach to living. Yoga is not merely a physical exercise. It can be used effectively to achieve personal peace and freedom and improve mental and physical well-being. The practice of yoga aims to overcome one's limitations of the body and offers the goal and the means to reach it.

PHILOSOPHY OF YOGA

Ancient seers, mystics, and sages used yoga over a period of more than 5,000 years to achieve harmony of body, mind, and spirit. This practice, which originated in India, consists of physical and mental disciplines that make us healthy, alert, and receptive. We can transform our perception of the world and the way we live in it. Yoga has grown and has been altered continuously through thousands of years to meet the changing conditions of humankind. It has always been directed toward allowing the individual to achieve his or her full potential as a human being and then to stretch beyond into spiritual consciousness.

The word "yoga" comes from the Sanskrit root *yug*, which means to yoke, bind, and unite. It implies harnessing oneself to a way of life or discipline to unite body, mind, and spirit. There are various branches of yoga such as Hatha yoga, Raja yoga, Juana yoga, Bhakti yoga, Mantra yoga, Laya yoga, and Tantric yoga. These branches are all closely interrelated. One cannot practice only one of these branches of yoga to the exclusion of the others. Practicing Hatha yoga may bring one naturally to involvement in Karma, Raga, or any other branch. The paths are interwoven so that the yoga practitioner aspires to merge knowledge and devotion while the body is kept as a healthy temple for the spirit. This chapter refers specifically to Hatha yoga, the branch that uses the physical body through the performance of asanas to channel the mind's energies. "Ha" and "Tha" are the Sanskrit syllables meaning sun and moon. They relate to the opposing forces in the universe: male-female, positive-negative, passive-aggressive. By balancing and reconciling these forces, one hopes to achieve serenity and wholeness. Hatha yoga may be an attractive path for one who enjoys a physical challenge to cultivate the body and mind.

The historical background of yoga is mainly in the Hindu tradition. When Yogis have achieved Samadi, or cosmic consciousness, it is interpreted in Hindu terms as contact with Brahama, the Universal Spirit. Yoga is not a religion and does not demand adherence to any one dogma. Anyone of any religion can be a yogi. Yoga is a technique of personal development that existed long before any system of philosophy. It has been used for health and healing as well. The simplest way to discover yoga is to practice it. In this way, you can recognize the many faces and ideas as they are described in such historic books as the Vedas, the Upanishads, the Mahabharata, the Bhagavadgita, and the yoga Sutras. These texts bring spiritual awareness and guidance to the life of the sadhaka (spiritual seeker) so that daily life can be faced and lived with courage and right action.

The yoga Sutras compiled and systematized by the Hindu sage Patanjali summarize yogic philosophy, principles, and practices. The Sutras, or threads, are condensed phrases that are clear, concise, and full of meaning. Passed on by an oral tradition to maintain the purity of knowledge, they were eventually put into writing. Many translations and interpretations of these exist. The yoga Sutras are composed of four chapters or Padas: (I) Samadi Pada describes the concept and essence of yoga. (II) Sadana Pada expounds on the practices that prepare the aspirant (sadhaka), physically and mentally. (III) Vibhuti Pada discusses how yogic powers (siddhis) are acquired. (IV) Kaivalya Pada explains the steps to final liberation from the limitations of human life. Patanjali gives guidelines for living a life of minimized stress and practical outlook. These basic guidelines are called Ashtanga yoga, meaning the "eight limbs." (Today, Ashtanga yoga has a totally different meaning that has nothing to do with classical yoga.) The eight steps to union with God are 1) ethical disciplines (yama); 2) rules of conduct (niyama); 3) physical discipline and posture (asana); 4) control of breath and subtle energy (pranayama); 5) withdrawal of the senses and internalization of the mind (pratyahara); 6) concentration (dharana); 7) meditation (dhyana); and 8) superconscious (self-realization or samadhi).

Yoga encompasses a set of ethical principles and moral precepts including diet, exercise, and meditative aspects based on the yamas and niyamas. The yamas are the ethical disciplines observed toward others in everyday life. The niyamas are rules of conduct that bring discipline to our lives by observing and practicing these two components of Ashtanga yoga. Disturbances of the mind and body are reduced and eventually eliminated. One can destroy the impurities of the body and mind and attain inner peace and happiness. Good health results from equilibrium of physical and emotional well-being.

YOGA THERAPY

If you have trouble relaxing and your body is stiff and aching or if you have frequent headaches, chronic neck, shoulder, or low back pain, yoga may be for you. Yoga has been used by both Eastern and Western medicine to treat various medical problems and to enhance health. Yoga's system of healing is based on the premise that the body may be allowed to function as naturally as possible. The yogic view of health and disease is unique. It looks at the human system as a comprehensive structure consisting of different layers of which the physical body is only a part. Yoga suggests that suffering may appear in one particular layer but might affect others. It suggests the need to go beyond dealing with symptoms.

A sequence of yoga asanas (postures) is recommended according to the ailment and physical and emotional condition of the patient. This has to be done under the guidance of a teacher (guru) who has the knowledge, training, and understanding of the asanas and their effects on the body system. If the sequence is inappropriate, more harm than good can be done. It is recommended that the treatment be carried out under the direction of an experienced teacher. Effectiveness of the cure depends upon the type of ailment, its progression, the patient's constitution, and commitment to the treatment. Yoga therapy is based on selecting and sequencing a series of asanas that stretch specific parts of the body and block others. In many cases, depending upon the nature of the problem, some of the suffering associated with the condition can be alleviated. Serious conditions can be more complicated and may take much longer to improve and recover. The patient can be active in the healing process and can be motivated to participate in the healing.

YOGA IN THE WEST

Yoga asanas along with meditation have become popular in the West, and yoga has become "Westernized." Postures are taught as ends in themselves to heal an illness, to reduce stress, or to look better. Yoga is thought of as calisthenics and sweat workouts. No longer placed in its classical context, yoga has taken on contemporary meanings. Large numbers of Americans are practicing yoga for its proposed health benefits, or because it is popular and well advertised and marketed. Tapes, videos, books, lines of clothing, food supplements, and furniture are all sold in the name of yoga. Many health professionals are referring their patients to yoga teachers for help in managing stress-related ailments and other physiological disorders. Yoga is regarded as a holistic approach to health that not only increases flexibility, strength, and stamina but also fosters self-awareness and peace of mind. It has become a household word in the West, and millions of men and women attend yoga classes, seminars, and yoga vacations and perform the physical exercises for which yoga is famous. Clearly, yoga is alive and flourishing in Western society today. Many people believe that this is yoga and are unaware of the totality of yoga as a philosophy of life.

Hatha yoga, the yoga of activity, is the path that most Westerners follow. There are various styles of Hatha yoga, and each has specific characteristics that reflect a particular teacher's approach to yoga asanas, such as Iyengar, Kundalini, Kripalu, Bikram, Sivanda, and others. Iyengar, a popular style in the West, is based on the teachings of living yoga master BKS Iyengar. The method is orderly and progressive. Postures are adjusted to the needs and physical conditions of the student necessary to take the body to the pose. (This author is a student and teacher of the Iyengar method of yoga and has tested this method.)

CLINICAL STUDIES ON THE PRACTICE OF YOGA

The practice of yoga has been credited for everything from reversing heart disease, alleviating symptoms of menopause, and treating and preventing osteoarthritis. It may also be another way of managing chronic ailments and easing chronic pain. People suffering from chronic pain go through more than just pain itself. They contend with depression, anxiety, and medication usage. A study conducted in California found that volunteers suffering from chronic pain from migraines and osteoarthritis, after combining meditative breathing techniques (known as pranayama) with yoga asanas, asked their physicians to decrease the dosages of their medications. Thus, yoga was effective in relieving pain.

A variety of yoga books have included specific recommendations for the treatment of various kinds of arthritis. The beneficial effects can be attributed to stretching, extending, and relaxing creating calmness of the mind. Gurus are quoted as saying that root causes of diseases can be identified and treated, not only symptoms and signs.

Accessible information is available about how the Iyengar method of Hatha yoga can be used as a supplement to other measures to treat musculoskeletal problems. Standing postures can strengthen and align the bones and muscles. Traction and active alignment from the use of your own muscles, if tolerated, may be preferable to passive traction by using external postures.

Regimens derived from the Iyengar method of Hatha yoga are described in some books for various types of physical and mental problems, including stress and pain. (See "Suggested Readings" on page 267.) While no real scientific documentation is available yet, there are countless testimonials of those who have benefited from these programs. The ailment will determine the method to be used, and details and illustrations provide this information. For example, yoga for knee problems addresses alignment, flexibility, and blood flow in the virasana cycle; the ankles, knees, and hips must be properly aligned to rest the legs and knees. For specific metabolic diseases like gout, no exercises should be done during acute attacks. Yoga therapy can be used during asymptomatic phases and is said to help dissolve deposits of uric acid in the lining of the joint, provided the damage is within a certain degree.

Yoga has received little objective evaluation. However, references to open studies have been found in asthma, hypertension, pain management, and mood. One study observed reduction of blood pressure with yoga, but no follow-up controlled study was to be found. Hatha yoga relaxation did slow breathing rate in chronic heart failure, reduced dyspnea (difficulty breathing), and reportedly produced an improvement in pulmonary gas exchange and exercise performance. In the rheumatic diseases, the two small controlled studies this author has conducted seem to be the only examples. Both of these employed the Iyengar method of Hatha yoga described above.

In osteoarthritis of the fingers, this author designed and conducted an Iyengar-based ten-week yoga program in which the intervention group received stretching and strengthening exercises emphasizing upper-body extension and alignment. The yoga group showed significant decrease in pain and tenderness and improved range of motion. More recently, this author designed and evaluated a program of Iyengar yoga and relaxation techniques that offered an effective treatment alternative for patients with carpal tunnel syndrome. Yoga was proposed to be helpful as stretching may relieve compression in the carpal tunnel, better joint posture may decrease intermittent compression, and blood flow may be improved to the median nerve. Four weeks after the conclusion of the program, the yoga group reported that they maintained improvement in their carpal tunnel symptoms. Further studies are needed to pursue the long-term effects of yoga on the painful symptoms of carpal tunnel syndrome and patient discomfort.

In the Iyengar system of Hatha yoga, the student is asked to work within simple well-defined abilities to direct conscious energy to specific sites of his or her own body-mind. Consciousness is subjective (of the mind), while energy is objective (of the body).

Together they form a mind-body union capable of generating and clarifying knowledge. Students use this as a "probe" to systematically contact all parts of the body-mind field. By the precise placement of the body parts and their activities in the postures (asanas), the pupil is able to generate specific vectors of energy, matter, awareness, and intention. Hopefully, there will be a growing awareness and broadening and deepening integration of body and mind. The student or patient can work to the capacity of his or her ability and gain clarity, awareness, and self-help. Under the direction of a capable and competent teacher, the student can begin to understand the depth and potential of an asana.

The results of this effort are evident in the growing numbers of yoga pupils in the United States and in the rest of the world. A person's whole being, engaged in yoga, can blossom and become pain and disease free. One can become stronger in order to handle other challenges of life. Many physicians, scientists, lawyers, homemakers, athletes, women and men of other professions, and even children have benefited for almost three decades from yoga taught by this author. Having traveled to India as a student, medical patient, and researcher of the method of yoga, this author is convinced that yoga is an effective way to treat and prevent traumatic pain.

THE EFFECTS OF YOGA

When the mind is stilled and the body relaxed, there is lightness, health, steadiness, and overall well-being. Yoga isn't in the medical mainstream yet, but some physicians are advising their patients to take yoga classes. Many find that yoga can be an important part of a successful treatment program. In the case of carpal tunnel syndrome, or even low back pain, surgery may be necessary in some cases, but yoga may be a favorable option.

Benefits of yoga can start with pain relief, but go much further. For one thing, yoga can ease the anxiety that often accompanies pain. It can bring order to chaos. When everything around you is crumbling, yoga helps you find peace within yourself and provides inner strength. Yoga teaches you to have a positive attitude and to do what you can for yourself. You don't have to run and get an operation right away. Through yoga, patients can gain a beneficial sense of control over their bodies. They can learn to breathe and relax. This is crucial for the reduction of pain.

On any given day, millions of Americans take pills to relieve headaches, neck and back pain, and/or stress-related aches and pains. Many end up taking drugs daily to deal with the effects of chronic pain, post-traumatic or otherwise. Even worse are the potential negative side effects related to this daily routine. The practice of yoga is noninvasive and empowering. You can develop a positive attitude and let pain be your teacher. You can take charge and manage your pain, as well as relieve symptoms of anxiety and depression. Whatever tools we use to counter illness, it is our attitude toward the whole process of healing that can reduce our suffering.

CONTRAINDICATIONS AND PRECAUTIONS

Yoga asanas done incorrectly or without preparation or supervision may cause disease and may contribute to other problems. For people with arthritis, asanas should be developed slowly when the joints or the spine is stiff. Depending upon the nature of the post-traumatic pain, a particular asana sequence must be carefully thought out. There is a variety of approaches to yoga and a high variation among yoga practitioners who are willing to offer yoga-based approaches to treatment. Asanas are based on human postures of standing, sitting, and lying down. They are not a series of movements to be followed mechanically. The postures have a logic that must be internalized if they are to be practiced correctly. The teacher must know the structure of the asana and know how to arrange the anatomical body of the patient, especially the limbs. The body is then molded to fit the structure of the asana. There must be no undue stress on any organ, muscle, bone, or joint.

Some examples of these systems mentioned earlier are Kundalini yoga developed by Yogi Bhajan; Kripalu developed by Yogi Amrit Desai and characterized by an internally directed approach to asana practice; Bikram yoga or "Hot Yoga" developed by Bikram Choudhury in which room temperature is at least 80°F or higher, and poses are done vigorously; integral yoga developed by Swami Satchidananda in which a set pattern of gentle meditative stretches, relaxing, and breathing is followed and ends with meditation; and Ashtanga vinyasa yoga developed by K. Pattabhi Jois—not to be confused with the eightfold path or Ashtanga yoga—that involves a vigorous, intensive set sequences of poses and is physically demanding to create heat—or tapas "to burn."

Iyengar yoga is Hatha yoga practiced in a manner prescribed by yoga master BKS Iyengar. It is probably the most widely recognized approach to Hatha yoga in the West. It is precise and dynamic. Close attention is paid to the placement of feet, hands, and pelvis and to the alignment of the spine, arms, and legs. Standing poses are emphasized, and after the student gains a certain proficiency with the postures, pranayama is taught. Iyengar has developed yoga props—blocks, benches, bolster, straps, and ropes—to aid a support system to achieve greater extension and ability in the posture. These aids are useful for students who are weak, stiff, or have various medical ailments. The final posture is achieved when all the parts of the body are positioned correctly with awareness and intelligence. Iyengar is recognized for his profound knowledge and development of the therapeutic applications of yoga.

How to pick a yoga consultant is even less clear than how to pick a doctor. Some certification is available, but there is little agreement as to what this means. For most people with arthritis or post-traumatic pain, depending on its nature, a more conservative, gradual approach to the poses seems most sensible. Done correctly, yoga can have a beneficial effect on the whole body. Asanas can tone muscles, tissues, ligaments, and joints, and also maintain functioning and health of the body's systems. The body and mind can be relaxed as yoga enhances recovery from fatigue and stress of daily living. With continued practice, you can experience the joy of the benefits of yoga.

Studies suggest that yoga might work in the treatment of osteoarthritis of the knee by fully extending the knee and strengthening the quadriceps. Various props such as ropes, wooden blocks, and belts can be used to enhance stretching the muscles. Beyond clinical observations, there is a growing amount of information suggesting that mechanical actions can have physiologic effects at the cellular level. Resultant changes in cell function are just beginning to be understood. Effects of mechanical and fluid pressure on structures, such as cartilage, also suggest that yoga postures might improve joint function. In experimental settings, good joint motion can preserve cartilage that is lost by immobilization. To avoid joint abuse and pain, a correctly supervised yoga program may be one way to provide motion and forces on joints needed to preserve integrity.

Remember, not all yoga is the same, and how to select an appropriate class or instructor as previously mentioned is not clear. Many Western-oriented presentations about yoga seem to make extravagant, inappropriate claims and should signal great caution. Unless something is documented, careful consumers should stick with yoga concepts that fit our physiologic understanding. Programs that gradually build from supervised and safe asanas seem reasonable. Those that make extravagant claims without documentation should be looked at carefully. Today, there is a tremendous interest in health consciousness. Many answers may be found in therapies such as yoga. Conventional medicine often is not adequate to help people gain physical fitness and mental poise. People are looking for natural, less invasive approaches to better health and pain relief. Yoga is practiced everywhere and is earning a place in the medical system for its therapeutic value. Through a therapeutic approach of a few basic asanas and pranayama, physical and mental well-being becomes possible. Yoga can tap the wisdom of the body to bring health to the surface.

YOGA TODAY

Most people who take up yoga in the West today do so for countless reasons. Yoga is fun, popular, and accessible. It is everywhere. There are yoga vacations, yoga trips, yoga food supplements, yoga camps, lines of yoga clothing, yoga supplies, and just about yoga everything. Rather than seeking the spiritual, one may turn to yoga to relax or just to have fun. Yoga postures are a marvelous method of physical exercise and relaxation. Soon it becomes apparent that physical tension is closely related to mental tension. Performing the postures demands concentration and stilling of the mind. You must concentrate in order to do them, as certain physical postures are expressive of mental states. A simple example is the reflection of mental tension in a tense neck, head, and shoulders.

Yoga stresses the relationships between all things rather than the divisions. It reflects everything in the environment just as the shape of objects is defined by the space around them. Every breath, every action, every thought reflects the environment. Many people see themselves as small separate units in an alien world, clinging to their identity and feeling helplessly insignificant. Their perception is colored by personal desires, anxieties, and prejudices. They do not see things clearly in a unified sense. Yoga can help clear the mind of egocentric thoughts and emotions. By learning to look and accept without judgment, one becomes receptive to the true nature of things, including one's self, and sees the world and those in it as a harmonious whole.

Pain is a normal part of life, but not a state in which to remain. Historically, benefits of yoga have been known for helping and healing. Practicing yoga may even end pain and provide a state of well-being.

Yoga is the antidote to the "rat race." It is noncompetitive. Each person knows his or her own achievements and abilities and is not to be judged by external standards. In yoga, there can be no failure as long as there is trying. According to Patanjali, "Success is immediate where effort is intense." One can start yoga anywhere and benefit from it. Yoga is not simply a means to an end, but a way of life.

While there can be no doubt that certain varieties of prescribed drugs have significantly contributed to the general welfare of humankind, there are many who feel that modern society is becoming overly reliant upon pharmaceuticals. While they remain one of the most effective forms of therapeutic treatment for many types of disease and post-traumatic pain, they have little in the way of preventive powers. Most experts agree that out of ignorance we abuse and neglect ourselves for half of our lives and then react with indignation, surprise, or grief when we find ourselves with ailments, aches, stiffness, and arthritis. In many cases, choosing an alternative therapy such as yoga could decrease and perhaps eliminate the need for prescribed medication.

Yoga keeps one healthy since it helps respiration, digestion, elimination, and circulation. It keeps the body supple, stretches the spine, and strengthens the muscles. Minor aliments and psychosomatic symptoms often disappear. You become more aware of your surroundings since yoga stimulates the entire organism. You feel more "alive." Whatever a person's problem—overeating, smoking, compulsive behaviors, pain, sadness—yoga can help by restoring the balance between the natural functions of the body and those of the mind. With regular practice, a person becomes in tune with him- or herself and may bring about personal life changes.

YOGA POSTURES (ASANAS)

Yoga postures are anatomically and physiologically sound. They guide the variety of movements attainable by the human body. In the Iyengar method of Hatha yoga, asanas have been categorized according to the level of difficulty from beginner to advanced student. The postures are grouped to the positioning of the body while standing, sitting, twisting, prone, supine, inverted, and balancing. (See figure 17.1 on page 264.) They incorporate slow and quick movement and stillness. Since the entire organic structure is invigorated and toned by practicing the postures, there are important therapeutic effects. Muscle tone is improved, and there is stamina and agility. (See figure 17.2 on page 264.)

On the psychological level, the postures are challenging and can "liven up" a lethargic and depressed person, or calm an anxious and distressed person. Yoga can heal parts of our bodies that have been injured and traumatized. It involves movements that stimulate injured parts of the body and also increases our ability to bear pain and or even reduce it. (See figure 17.3 on page 264.)

GUIDELINES FOR HATHA YOGA PRACTICE

Place and Time

Choose a clean quiet place in early morning or evening. In the morning, you may feel fresh and energetic but stiff. In the evening, you will feel looser but may be tired. Adjust accordingly. It is not advisable to practice on the sand or in the sun as the foundation is not firm and the heat of the sun is dehydrating.

Clothes and Equipment

Clothing should be completely unrestricting and allow bending and stretching. Feet should be bare to have freedom of movement and make firm contact with the floor or a non-slippery mat.

Food and Drink

Stomach, bladder, and bowels should be empty. Yoga should not be done for three or four hours after a main meal or for one hour after a light snack. If you are hungry, have a cup of coffee, tea, or milk a half-hour beforehand. Do not drink water during practice.

Consistent Practice

Try to practice daily for short, regular intervals. It is more rewarding to spend fifteen minutes each day practicing yoga than it is to practice once a week for two hours or to practice intensely for two to three days.

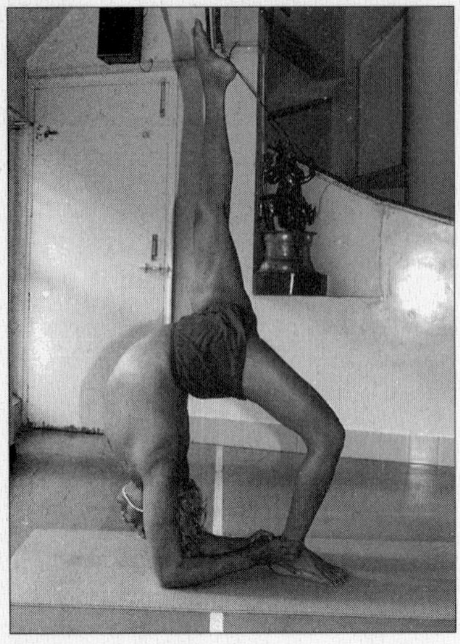

FIGURE 17.1
Asana (posture): Eka Pada Viparita Dandasna I (one leg pointed to ceiling). This pose tones the spine, extends the chest fully, and soothes the mind. (Photo printed with permission of BKS Iyengar.)

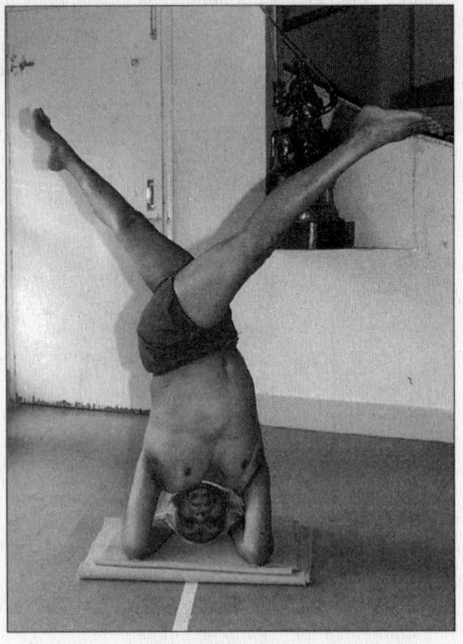

FIGURE 17.2
Asana (posture): Parivrttaikapada Sirsasana (headstand with legs spread and torso and legs turned). This pose develops the leg muscles and tones the kidneys, bladder, prostate, and intestines. (Photo printed with permission of BKS Iyengar.)

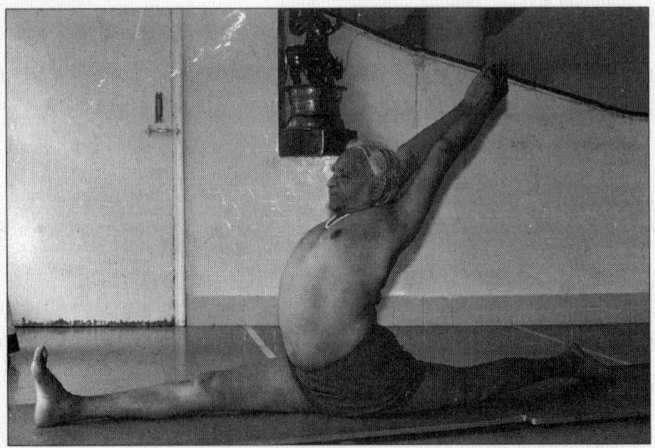

FIGURE 17.3
Asana (posture): Hanumanasana (split). This pose helps cure sciatica. It tones the leg muscles and strengthens the abductor muscles of the thighs. (Photo printed with permission of BKS Iyengar.)

Attitude

Find enjoyment in your practice and do not judge yourself if you are unable to do everything at once. Appreciate your body as it is in the moment. Think positively.

Attentiveness

One cannot practice only one branch of yoga to the exclusion of the others. Practicing Hatha yoga may bring one naturally to involvement in Karma, Raga, or any other branch. The paths are interwoven so that the yoga practitioner aspires to merge knowledge and devotion while the body is kept as a healthy temple for the spirit.

Awareness

Avoid overstretching. Pay attention to pain. It is an excellent teacher and will keep you alert to how your body responds. Keep your eyes open, but relax them and relax your ears as well. Relax your face and jaw.

Props

Chairs, walls, blankets, belts, ropes, or blocks are used to facilitate the stretches. Using a chair is helpful for people who are stiff, injured, or fatigued. Using props can bring one's body to fullest extension. They are not "crutches" but aids in taking the body to the pose. Props are meant to be used as interim help and can be set aside later.

Yoga poses differ from exercise as they consist of moving into a position and holding it. Often, they are synchronized with breathing and work every part of the body including fingers and joints, internal organs, glands, and circulatory and respiratory systems. They are designed to restore the body to its original flexibility, allowing full range of movement. Some postures are relaxed, others are dynamic and strenuous. Be aware of your limitations and never force your body into a position.

Breathing

Always breathe through your nose if possible. Normally, a movement requiring effort is done on an exhalation with a deep inhalation before it. Never hold your breath. Let your breath work with your body. Breathing deeply and freely will help your body ease into postures. Inhale when using upward, opening, expanding movements away from the body. Exhale when twisting and closing movements toward the center of the body are used.

Cautions

Start slowly. It is better to repeat movements two or three times than to hold a position. These poses should feel comfortable. Adjustments may need to be made. Stop if there is undue strain in the face, ears, or eyes or in breathing.

People with heart conditions, high or low blood pressure, detached retina, recent surgery, or any special abnormal condition should check with a doctor, as should pregnant women. Remember that there are beneficial postures for almost every condition, but some should be avoided at special times. Women should not practice inverted poses during menstruation.

After every yoga session, one should relax in savasana (corpse position) for a few minutes for relaxation, recuperation, and reward. Sources for directions for savasana are provided in the Suggested Readings.

GUIDELINES FOR FINDING A TEACHER AND STYLE OF YOGA

- Know the credentials of the teacher, and the training and style of yoga being taught. Teacher training and certification vary widely.
- Discuss with the teacher what you are looking for.
- Take classes in different styles to find which one appeals to you. Classes vary from teacher to teacher and style to style.
- Make certain your teacher knows of your ailments and is qualified to help. Remember, yoga teachers are not doctors. If necessary, get your doctor's permission.
- Stick with one method once you have found a style with which you are comfortable.

THE EFFECT of the asanas on the mind is relaxing. In the words of BKS Iyengar, "It is the body alone which should be active while the brain should remain passive, watchful and alert." Yoga is not a cure-all for everything that ails you. If practiced diligently and with commitment, it may make a major and even profound difference in your life.

SUGGESTED READINGS

Iyengar, B.K.S. *Light on Pranayama.* New York: Crossroad Publishing, 1981.

A practical guide to the yogic art of breathing.

———. *Light on Yoga.* New York: Shocken Books, 1979.

A classical text on the philosophy and practice of yoga.

———. *Yoga: The Path to Holistic Health.* London: Dorling Kindersley, 2001.

Iyengar, Geeta S. *Yoga: A Gem for Women.* New Delhi: Allied Publishers Private Limited, 1985.

Detailed description of yoga benefits and therapeutic application for women.

Mehta, Silva, Mira, and Shyam. *Yoga the Iyengar Way.* New York: Alfred A. Knopf, 1990.

HELPFUL WEB SITES

BKS Iyengar
http://bksiyengar.com

Lists certified teachers and yoga schools.

Yoga International
http://www.yimag.org

Online magazine lists directories of teachers and yoga schools.

Yoga Journal
http://www.yogajournal.com

Online magazine lists directories of teachers and yoga schools.

18

Disability versus Impairment

BARRY SNYDER, M.D.

Medicine has progressed to effectively treat many illnesses that were once beyond our control. Some disabling ailments were considered hopeless conditions for those people afflicted by them. Many examples illustrate the ability to ameliorate or eliminate a condition when it can be identified and a treatment regimen made available. Consider, for example, smallpox, tuberculosis, polio, or AIDS. Smallpox was virtually cured by immunization. Tuberculosis was once considered incurable. Now, if treated early, relatively few aftereffects remain following antibiotic therapy. Some individuals may remain disabled—particularly if treatment was delayed. In that event, they will experience physical limitations. Modifications to their lifestyles and surroundings will follow in accordance with those limitations. Polio was eradicated by vaccination. Physical treatment, adaptations, and psychosocial intervention have allowed victims who suffer residual impairment due to polio or post-polio syndrome to productively function as an integral part of society. AIDS is still a terminal illness, but quality and quantity of life have improved because of effective pharmaceutical treatment. Legal rights of these individuals have been protected from discrimination arising out of prejudices and misconceptions about the disease. Support groups assist individuals to cope with personal and cultural interactions associated with the illness, thereby lessening their sense of isolation.

Aside from infectious diseases, there are many conditions that once doomed those who were affected by them to a lifetime of dependency and, in some cases, isolation. Trauma centers have developed into multi-specialty facilities that have saved lives and limbs that were once given up as unsalvageable. Prosthetic designs have enabled many people to remain self-sufficient after the loss of one or more extremities. Pharmaceutical developments in rheumatology have helped remit the progression of some types of arthritis. Orthopedic surgical procedures have been developed to replace badly affected joints and to restore function to close to normal.

If you suffer from a chronic pain disorder and do not have an actual "disease" like those mentioned, you might ask how this relates to you. Actually, it is not very different. For reasons that we shall discuss, treatment of pain—specifically, chronic pain—has also advanced. Diagnostic acumen and therapeutic methods have improved. Newer pharmaceuticals and newer, more comprehensive procedural techniques and approaches have been developed. As a result, pain management has become a subspecialty involving several disciplines. Injection therapy and medications are prescribed to control pain in its early stages. Should residual impairment be recognized at the conclusion of that treatment, current and future needs within the environment in which that person will function are established. When necessary, and if feasible, the surroundings can be physically changed to adjust to those needs, accordingly. If appropriate, assistive devices may be provided to adapt to the demands of daily living and facilitate return to maximum function. Medications may still be prescribed, but they may differ from the early prescriptions by types and quantities.

IDENTIFYING THE PROBLEM

The starting point must be identification of the problem. It may be an illness or injury associated with pain or a primary pain disorder. For the former, pain is a secondary result of the underlying condition. Consider, as an example, a compound fractured limb that is complicated by a chronic infection of the bone (osteomyelitis) and does not heal. Pain of varying degrees will continue until the fracture is healed and the infection is eliminated or suppressed. The primary pain disorder, such as reflex sympathetic dystrophy or fibromyalgia, as far as we know, is characterized by a condition of pain with secondary physical and psychological manifestations. Pain becomes the disease, rather than a result of it. These have been recently classified by the American Medical Association as complex regional pain syndromes.

It is not always possible to identify a cause of chronic pain, since there are some conditions that are not clearly defined. In most cases, however, diagnoses can be made—even if it is for a disease process that is associated with pain in some unknown way. Identification, to the extent that it can be made, will give some direction for treatment. Patients tend to be more accepting if they can label their plan. It is authenticated if they can respond to a question about it with an "official" diagnosis. As we shall see, it is equally important to recognize that too much emphasis can be given to the diagnosis. If allowed, it might create or perpetuate passive-dependent behavior that can become counterproductive to treatment. Physical treatment is initiated, based on that clinical impression, just as any other disease entity. Once the treatment has been completed, residual chronic pain and any physical handicap associated with the disability are addressed. When the pain occurs after injury (trauma), it may be called post-traumatic pain or fall within the category of post-traumatic pain disorders. Extended treatment is the same as it would be for any other residual impairment and the individual it affects.

UNDERSTANDING CHRONIC PAIN DISORDERS

A few concepts should be described if we are to understand an extended course of management for the chronic pain disorder. First, let us define acute versus chronic. The simplest of definitions differentiates the two in terms of time. An acute condition is one that has recently occurred. The biomedical model of treatment is applicable to the acute problem. It is primarily approached by physical means, although there may be secondary psychological or cultural effects that must be dealt with. This treatment may include medication, hospitalization, or surgery.

A chronic disorder has classically been defined as one that continues for a protracted period of time—perhaps six months or more. Because of our clinical experiences within the medical and allied professions over the years, we have become more sensitized to the secondary effects of a chronic condition. Consequently, greater emphasis is given to the psychosocial consequences that characterize the chronic pain disorder. The model used to treat it would appropriately be termed biopsychosocial rather than biomedical. Acute pain may be associated with an underlying visceral injury or illness, such as a fracture, appendicitis, or tumor. It usually responds to treatment of its cause and analgesic medication until that treatment is completed. Chronic pain, on the other hand, continues after this initial treatment.

Persistence of pain as part of a chronic pain syndrome may not have a clear explanation. Therefore, the effects of chronic pain and its causes distinguish it from the acute condition by more than a temporal relationship.

Often, patients suffering from a chronic pain disorder may develop symptoms that exceed physical explanation. This is part of the psychology involved with chronic pain. It is not unusual for patients to pass from one physician to another in search of a diagnosis. The provider offers treatment only to subsequently disappoint the patient with the all-too-common response "you'll have to live with it" when it becomes evident that there has been no substantial lasting change. Inordinate reliance on medications, deterioration of personal relationships, loss of self-esteem, and depression. These are some of the problems that need to be addressed during long-term management of chronic pain.

Chronic pain may also be distinguished as either malignant or nonmalignant. It may be reasonable to refer to a chronically painful condition as a chronic pain syndrome, if it is not due to a malignancy. Even though pain of a malignant condition may be protracted and incapacitating, there is a distinction. A chronic pain syndrome may be the primary illness itself, rather than secondary to another illness that is clearly definable. Nonmalignant chronic pain is not likely to have a defined period of duration, whereas pain occurring because of malignancy usually has some endpoint defined by the primary disease.

IMPAIRMENT VERSUS DISABILITY

The distinction between impairment and disability should be understood. In part, this a legal issue. Medical providers determine the extent to which body function has been lost by physical examination and testing. The court system and its social agencies will apply that information to the daily needs for, and limits of, the settings in which the disabled person conducts activities of living. Ranges of motion, strength, and other obvious physical parameters primarily defined physical capabilities at one time. Over the years, assessment of impaired function has become more elaborate. This is most evident in the guidelines published by the American Medical Association. Function is evaluated by specific findings on physical examination that are compared with those that are expected. A compendium of the normal values has been listed in the AMA's Guides to the Evaluation of Permanent Impairment. Based on a specific diagnosis or injury, a value is given that represents the percentage by which the extremity, region, or entire body function is reduced from its whole value.

However, two people with the same impairment may be affected in entirely different ways. Though impairment becomes the foundation for disability determination, the two are not synonymous. For example, a bus driver who loses a finger would be disabled from work in an entirely different way than would a musician with the very same injury and the same level of impairment. Notwithstanding work requirements, two individuals with the same impairment may have entirely different social situations that, because of the daily demands for activities of living, may require different levels of physical function or capability to meet those demands. Consequently, disability is a much larger issue for which impairment is only a component.

Psychological, social, occupational, and cultural influences play significant roles in determining disability. The interplay between the individual and his or her environment is dynamic. Many disciplines will assess the degree to which residual impairment resulting from chronic pain and injury, if applicable, restricts that person's ability to function within the physical demands imposed by work, home, and the social setting. Only after the input by all of these professionals has been analyzed will some determination of disability be made. Usually, it is left to the court system to reach a conclusion as to the overall disability. This may be through mediation within the insurance industry, an arbitration panel, a worker's compensation referee, the Social Security Department of Disability Determination, or a civil court. In any case, it is not just the pain, injury, and physical loss but a much broader view of the interactions resulting from that impairment that must be considered for disability.

Albert's Story of Impairment

Albert works in a supermarket. He is constantly on his feet and must walk in and out of a refrigeration unit. After a work-related incident, he developed incapacitating low back pain radiating to his right buttock and thigh. Recognition of his problem and the ultimate diagnosis was delayed because of a prior history of back and leg pain for which he had undergone operative treatment years earlier. His left leg was involved at that time, and there were complications from the surgery. When all of the diagnostic studies were completed, it became evident that his acute symptoms were due to herniation of an intervertebral disc at an entirely different level from the one that had herniated more than fifteen years earlier. He was fearful of undergoing another operation on his back because of the prior complications. Nonoperative measures of treatment were undertaken, leading to relief of many of his symptoms. He reached a point at which he was much more comfortable, but residual physical impairment resulting from the recent disc herniation remained. The situation presented a conflict for Albert. Impairment from the old back problem never limited him from the work he had been doing for years before the current event. He wanted to return to work, but he knew the physical activities required for his job were probably beyond his capabilities because of the recent injury and the new limitations caused by it. Furthermore, some treatment was needed for residual pain.

MOST OF YOU who are reading this are probably able to relate to Albert's story because you have gone through it or know someone who has. In many cases, patients are told there is nothing more that can be done and they just have to live with the pain. There was once a time when that was accepted practice and not much more could be offered. Without an understanding of the chronic pain patient, that remains the way of thinking. Many are written off because no clear cause for their pain can be found. Others may seem to have a reason for pain, but the extent of their complaints exceeds the expected levels. Professionals may summarily dismiss them as having complaints that are in their heads. Unknowingly, they may have stated a major attribute of the problem, but they fail to recognize it. Having it "in your head" occurs for a reason. The interplay of physical and emotional must be tackled. More often than not, the underlying problem escapes complete delineation because of ignorance and too little effort by the physician(s) or other providers.

BIOMEDICAL APPROACH TO PAIN MANAGEMENT

Pain management can deal with the physical aspects of pain by administering physical treatment. This is called the biomedical approach. It can be administered at different levels of sophistication. In a clinical setting, medications are prescribed. At a slightly greater level, clinics have been established through which injection therapy can be given. This includes epidural corticosteroid injections, trigger-point injections, facet blocks, and sympathetic nerve blocks. Injection therapy is more reasonably given during the acute phase of treatment. For most patients, by the time they have reached a stage of chronic pain, those modalities have been utilized with limited or no beneficial effect. Care should be given to avoid fostering a dependency on them. It becomes too easy to rely on those methods in which you play a relatively passive role. Ablative therapy may be another level of treatment offering relief that is more lasting. Rhizotomy is the technical term for this procedure. It is usually done with a form of high-frequency energy waves (radio frequency similar to microwave) that causes temperature to increase at a segment of the nerve called the dorsal root ganglion. It may be of value for arthritic joints of the spine. Theoretically, without those nerves that carry pain sensation, pain does not occur. As good as it sounds, it does not always work as effectively. When it does, relief may be only temporary.

HOLISTIC PAIN MANAGEMENT

Fortunately, the road does not end at the point at which standard biomedical methods of treatment are no longer effective. Holistic pain management, as a subspecialty, involves input from multiple disciplines—

internal medicine, physiatry, orthopedic surgery, neurology, neurosurgery, psychology, psychiatry, social service, occupational therapy, physical therapy, vocational counseling, and the list goes on. It will take a great deal on your part, but resources are available to treat your chronic pain symptoms even after you have reached an apparent plateau. Once this level has been identified, evaluation and management can begin within a multidisciplinary pain-management center. We will discuss the process of holistic pain management for the remainder of this chapter.

Coming to Grips with Your Pain

First and foremost, a person suffering from chronic pain—be it a complex regional pain syndrome or a chronic pain syndrome that results from some other disorder—must come to grips with it. Facing the real fact that you have a pain disorder that may not be cured is essential to effective treatment. Denial becomes a normal response to this situation, and it must be overcome. Once you have accomplished the difficult task of realizing that reality, treatment may become much simpler. Rather than dwelling on the negative aspects of their disabilities, I encourage my patients to meet their illness and impairments head-on. From that point forward, having accepted their physical limitations, we can analyze aspects of their daily life and assess whether or not they are capable of working within those limits. Instead of summarily dismissing an activity by saying, "I can't," we look at this situation and say, "Can I?"

Attitude Recognition

When you have a cold or fever, you might feel quite miserable. Can you imagine what it would be like if those symptoms continued in perpetuity? Well, that is just an inkling of what some people experience with chronic pain. After a time, it takes its toll. Each day becomes a chore. Work becomes burdensome. Personal relationships become strained. Family, friends, and business associates distance themselves from you. If allowed to continue, the extreme consequences are disenfranchisement—loss of companionship, unemployment, loss of self-esteem, and despair. As you become increasingly estranged, you tend to withdraw even more. Bitter at what you perceive to be your ultimate plight, you draw attention to yourself by manipulating your environment to your needs by emphasizing your pain. The result is called pain behavior. People cater to you because you portray this helplessness. Yet they may resent your untiring complaints as you continue to seek attention by this means.

The paradox is not that you cannot live with the pain; the behavior has become ingrained to the extent that you need the pain to continue to live. You learn that it is, seemingly, your most effective way to promote personal contact, even if it is self-destructive. As long as it continues, the cycle will persist. You manipulate your environment by making demands; people attend to you, but learn to avoid you; you become more isolated, angry, and depressed, leading to the same behavior. It is not to say you should feel guilty for feeling pain. On the contrary, part of the treatment is to realize you are entitled to have pain. The appropriate manner in which behavior becomes channeled, though, constitutes part of the extended treatment for chronic pain.

Attitude recognition should not be only your responsibility; it should also be the responsibility of your physician to understand your feelings about your pain. After all, unless your emotions are brought into the open by discussing them, they may not be appreciated. To overlook the way in which you perceive the pain syndrome, more of your treatment will be devoted to talking at you than talking with you. With discussion comes rapport; with rapport comes understanding; and with understanding comes change.

Physical Activity

Now you are ready to set goals for your rehabilitation. There is nothing wrong with aspiring to limits that will force you to reach for them. However, it is important that you do not set those limits too high for yourself. Many small steps will always be more effective than one large leap. You will be less likely to be overwhelmed and stumble. More important, you will be more likely to approach your objective. Then, the next goal can be taken a step higher. These are usually directed to specific tasks. Some will involve day-to-day activities. In most cases, those goals will be directed to work, since it is one fundamental group of activities that promotes a personal sense of worth and social interaction.

Physical activities are encouraged, all the while. Extension of pain management requires a biomedical (that is, a physically oriented) approach and a psychosocial approach. The two become inseparable because of the effect that the physical ailment has on one's circle of life. Conventional medical management used to dictate rest when someone experienced pain. That was employed for acute pain symptoms and extrapolated to chronic pain management. Over the past several decades, we have come to realize that activity plays an essential role in the rehabilitation—even recovery, at times—of the individual suffering with chronic pain. Physiologic effects of exercise prompt the release of chemical mediators that are produced in the brain to actually reduce pain. These substances—called endogenous analgesics—are potent organic compounds that are released into the circulation as activity levels increase. Among them are chemicals called endorphins and enkephalins. Significant levels of pain can be tolerated because of these naturally occurring analgesics whose production is stimulated by exercise. Adrenalinelike compounds also are released during exercise to increase our heart rate, improve our circulation, and heighten our physical response. We develop a "high" when performing certain levels of activity because of these internally produced chemical compounds. In response, our bodies are facilitated to perform at an enhanced level. Athletes produce high levels of these chemicals. In part, that is why they can attain and endure their level of physical activities.

Though prescriptions for narcotic analgesics—called opioids—are given with the best intentions, one of the adverse effects is that the body senses the presence of them in the circulation and stops producing its own analgesics. It mistakenly interprets this to mean a sufficient amount has been produced to acquire that level. As a result, the body's own chemicals that effectively decrease pain are secreted at a lower level or are no longer produced. More prescription pain medication is needed as a substitute.

With continued rest and inactivity, our bodies become deconditioned. Activity, on the other hand, promotes flexibility and strength to approach a more optimal level. Risk of a number of disease conditions can be reduced by exercise as well. These include heart disease, diabetes mellitus, osteoporosis, and muscle injury. Ordinarily, deconditioning presents a major problem for the majority of the American population. Only 20 percent of people report physical activity of at least thirty minutes per day for five or more days per week. The problems of limited motion, weakness, loss of endurance, and loss of tissue elasticity are reversed as exercise levels improve.

Physical Rehabilitation—Work-Hardening

Physical therapy is the conventional model used in rehabilitation. For the treatment of chronic pain, physical modalities—ultrasound, hot packs, cold therapy, electromuscular stimulation, to name a few—may be utilized, but a program of active participation should be emphasized. Incrementally more demanding objectives are formulated.

Before injury or onset of chronic pain symptoms, those of you who were employed interacted within the workplace. Skills utilized within that environment are carried outside of work. They are not only used in our vocations but are also utilized in day-to-day activities at home and during recreation. Of course, those exact activities may not be employed in the same manner or to the same extent when applied to recreational and other social settings, but, like limbs of a tree, they branch into our everyday lives. Work activities are often the parameters used in a conditioning program because they specifically apply to the predominant portion of daily life for those individuals who were, or still are, employed. This concept of goal-oriented rehabilitation is administered within what is termed a "working conditioning" or "work-hardening" regimen.

Work-hardening utilizes the job description of your previous employment. In it, activities are categorized as to whether they could be performed "occasionally," "frequently," or "constantly." These are terms used by the U.S. Department of Labor to designate the fraction of an eight-hour workday that is spent doing the respective physical activity. By definition, the term "occasionally" means the task or activity is performed up to 33 percent of the eight-hour workday. "Frequent" activity means it is done from 34 to 66 percent of the workday. For an activity to be "constant," it is performed 67 percent or more of the workday. Activities such as sitting, standing, walking, and driving may be defined in these terms for the entire workday. Additionally, a given number of hours can be noted for any of those activities to be done for an uninterrupted period before resting—the number of hours the activity is performed without a break. Other designated activities customarily include such things as bending, stooping, crawling, crouching, reaching, and balancing. Fine manipulation and gross manipulation of hand function are assessed, as is repetitive use of upper and lower extremities. Capacity for lifting or carrying weight is usually noted within a job description as well. Reaching activities will interact with these lifting requirements.

A comprehensive explanation will include lifting specific amounts of weight at certain levels of height. It usually includes lifting from floor to chair level, below or at waist level, above waist to shoulder level, and above shoulder level. Carrying differs from lifting in that it requires a weight to be horizontally moved from one position to another. In its classic definition, analogy is given to carrying a suitcase for a given distance.

Very often, a vocational counselor is assigned or chosen to help manage the rehabilitation process. Unfortunately, there are times when this person does not tap into the resources that are at his or her disposal. Fortunately, that is usually the exception. If a constructive professional relationship between the rehabilitation counselor, doctor, and patient is established, the course of treatment can be facilitated. He or she will help to arrange for placement in an appropriate rehabilitation facility. Though part of your mindset may have led you to distrust many people in this position, try to establish a rapport, and you may find that the relationship becomes a positive influence on your overall rehabilitation.

In the previous illustration, Albert's sincere desire to return to work was discussed, but there was a question of how much he was capable of doing. In order for Albert to begin his rehabilitation program, his employer was asked for a job description. At first, it was somewhat vague and did not describe his position in the details that were just noted. I reviewed it and discussed the tasks involved in his work with his case manager and employer, arriving at a reasonable description. Obviously, if he had never been able to frequently lift seventy-five pounds at waist level before his injury, it would be unreasonable to expect him to do so now. We were ready to proceed with his rehabilitation, once these objectives were posted. It did not mean that he would reach these ultimate goals. They were used because he had once demonstrated an ability to perform them.

Work-hardening should begin after referral and acceptance to an accredited program. To start off, it is also necessary to establish your present physical capabilities. This gives a reasonable idea of the level at which you are currently able to function and how much of a difference there is between your capabilities and those required for your return to full work activities. Several formats are available for functional capacity assessment. Familiar tests include the KEY Functional Capacity Assessment, Blankenship Functional Capacity Evaluation, and ERGOS Work Simulator. It is quite likely that you will not achieve all the activities necessary for your work. Knowing your baseline permits an objective assessment of your progress.

Consistency of performance is usually measured as a part of these assessments. It is hoped the effort that you put forth will demonstrate a valid representation of your capabilities at that time. To help ensure it, some degree of pain must be tolerated. The KEY assessment takes it a step further by describing the type of validity that is observed. If a test is "valid," it is a reasonable representation of your physical capabilities *at that time.* If your overall performance is consistent but some aspects of testing were not because you did not exert full effort, it is labeled "conditionally valid." When performance is consistent and the examinee pushes himself or herself beyond those limits, it is termed "conditionally invalid." It is an invalid representation insofar as appearing to show you are able to do more than your actual capabilities at that time. The distinction between valid and invalid earmarks whether or not it is safe to perform within the demonstrated levels. The "conditionally valid" individual is so-called because he or she is functioning at a level that is less than his or her limits, but he or she can validly perform those activities. The overachiever whose results are shown to be "conditionally invalid" could be injured if permitted to exercise at that level at that time, because he or she is exceeding his or her capacity. Last, an "invalid" result shows that performance has been without any reasonable consistency that would demonstrate a representative effort. They may include the person who is not being forthright or malingering. Those patients who are identified as "invalid" are not reasonable candidates for work-hardening. Do not be intimidated by this evaluation. Remember, it is a test of your present capabilities.

In Albert's case, he underwent a KEY Functional Capacity Assessment that showed his performance to be a valid representation of his capabilities. As anticipated, his job description substantially exceeded the activities and type of work he was capable of tolerating at the time the evaluation was completed. The vocational counselor, occupational therapist/physical therapist, and I conferred to outline a regimen to be followed and to reinforce the limits that were to be set as the goals of his rehabilitation. A letter was sent to his employer and insurance carrier to inform them that he was to begin this program of treatment and assessment. Attached with it were an explanation of work-hardening and the period of time it would be administered.

Tasks involved in the work environment are reproduced in work-hardening. Activities may be performed that do not seem to reproduce those done at work. Superficially, that may appear to be the case, but the intent is to simulate the predominant activities necessary to perform a task without necessarily reproducing them. Several participants are usually at the work-hardening facility, performing their prescribed programs at different workstations. At first, only a few hours are spent each day at these activities. You are treated as an employee—punching the time clock when you arrive, when you take a break, and when you leave. Daily time is progressively increased to a six- to eight-hour day, five days per week. Some patients may require only four weeks of treatment. They may have very specific impairments of a single limb or upper extremities and are usually at an advanced stage of rehabilitation that needs to be tweaked. The overwhelming majority of patients involved in work-hardening continue for approximately eight weeks. During that time, you will periodically return to your treating physician—perhaps once or twice—to monitor your clinical status. An occasional patient may be recognized as feeling overwhelmed and might benefit by resting for a day. That should be done *only* with the doctor's full knowledge and approval.

At the conclusion of work-hardening, the functional capacity evaluation is repeated. You are likely to experience discomfort at the completion of the assessment or by the next day, because you have been pushed to your physical limits. Under most circumstances, symptoms resolve within a few days. Comparison is made to the baseline evaluation to assess the extent to which capabilities have improved. Results of the final assessment are also matched against the job description that was provided to define your goals at the beginning. If they coincide, it is very likely you will be able to return to your previous occupation and job description. Infrequently, extenuating circumstances may delay or prevent you from returning. Commonly, patients who have a disorder associated with chronic pain—be it from a complex regional pain syndrome or secondary to an underlying injury or nonmalignant illness—will demonstrate improvement with some residual limitations that do not fully compare to their previous job description.

After completing the work-hardening protocol, Albert, his vocational counselor, and I discussed the results and compared those findings with the information provided by his employer. To no surprise, he was not able to perform some of the requirements for his work. In particular, periods of rest were necessary more often, rather than virtually standing throughout the workday. Occasionally lifting up to fifty pounds was necessary for his work as he performed it at the time of injury. Albert reached a lifting limit of about thirty to thirty-five pounds and a plateau at that point. A number of tested activities, such as crawling or repetitive use of his hands or lower extremities, were not necessary for his work. Other listed activities remained pretty much in keeping with his demonstrated physical capabilities. He was able to return to work after presenting a report of our opinions that were based on these results and our discussions. His employer provided accommodations by keeping him at those recommended limitations. Assistance was to be given whenever a situation would exceed his capabilities.

When the point is reached at which, to a degree of certainty, there is no further improvement, it is termed the "level of maximum medical improvement." Many of the agencies that rely on these tests look for this endpoint. Too often, completion of work-hardening is thought to represent maximum medical improvement. There are limitations to the functional capacity assessment, however. It is administered in a nonthreatening environment. The situation to which the employee will return may pose a more daunting venue. It is dependent on interaction with administration and fellow employees, physical provisions within the workplace, and the employee's motivation.

This last consideration plays an important role that is often overlooked or dismissed. The longer you experience pain without therapeutic intervention, the less likely will be your return to work, *if you let it happen.* A normal consequence of your sense of loss—aside from the problems of denial that we have already discussed—is anger. You may not be able to help yourself from becoming angry at a system that has been unable to cure you or support you up until now. You are simply angry because you are still in pain and it appears that no one believes you or cares. Hopefully, you have begun to realize that you are capable of performing more than you once thought and that you will be able to survive in spite of your pain. Much of what is done will not be to cure your pain but to teach you how to live with it. The whole concept of pain management involves coordination of your personal needs, your physical limitations, and the available resources that will enable you to cope and function with your chronic symptoms. Now you have identified your limitations and you can focus on your strengths. This cannot be accomplished unless there is a strong support group to help you develop and maintain a level of motivation that will keep you moving in a forward direction.

An example of the inadequacy of simply relying on results of work-hardening to determine the ability to return to a previous work environment is illustrated by a patient who had a positive outcome. Jerry is a police detective. While apprehending an assailant behind the wheel of a vehicle, his arm was abruptly pulled as the driver took off. Virtually all of his rotator cuff—the complex of tendons that move the shoulder joint—was ripped off its attachment. After undergoing an extensive operation to repair the injury, he began a physical therapy program. The point was reached at which he did not seem to progress any further. It appeared that the repair had adequately healed; so, he was enrolled in work-hardening. At its completion, most of the activities in his job description were within his physical capabilities. Because he was approaching sixty years old, he opted for an early retirement and began a new position as an instructor. Jerry had reached the age at which he felt it was time to slow down and avoid some of the risks that were inherent in his job that resulted in his injury.

Psychological Counseling

Before devoting additional discussion pertaining to the resources that may be used to bring you back to work, the other side of rehabilitation must be given equal consideration. Early in this chapter, the description of chronic pain was distinguished by the greater emphasis placed on psychosocial aspects of the disorder. Pain management, when administered from a holistic perspective, deals with physical modalities of treatment and the multidisciplinary approach to the psychosocial aspects as well—a biopsychosocial model, it was called. Psychological background on which your pain continues to be superimposed influences your perception and reaction to it. We all have good days and bad days. I know if I have already been upset by something and stub my toe, I would be more likely to yell out and use some choice off-color remarks. Why shouldn't someone who is chronically having pain react in a similar way? You are entitled to experience pain. The manner in which you react to the effects it imposes needs to be properly directed. That can be done with group counseling, psychological counseling, and other support systems. Here, the vocational counselor, your physician, and other providers can promote healthy interaction between you and your family and friends. Familial involvement with the chronic pain patient is important for several reasons. One is to convey an understanding of the pain and its limitations. Another is to break the passive dependent cycle of pain behavior by reinforcing interaction that is more appropriate. Attitudes must be changed in order to move in a positive direction. This is not a concept that can be treated in this short space and time. It has been mentioned because it is as important as any other aspect of your rehabilitation—if not *the* most important.

Stress considerably influences the emotional aspects of the chronic pain patient. Psychological counseling enables you to open up about these feelings. By doing so, you will not feel as isolated and your level of stress will decrease. Relaxation techniques can be learned as an adjunct to therapy. If you are more relaxed in the situation where you are discussing stressors, you will be more likely to continue that treatment. Furthermore, you associate these stressful conditions with relaxation techniques as a conditioning response. Biofeedback is used in this context and can be extended outside of the professional office. Exercises in relaxation are instructed to be followed at home, while driving your car, or when in a public place. It becomes learned behavior for your everyday life. With less stress and greater relaxation, your pain becomes less overwhelming.

Aside from the physical performance demonstrated in work-hardening, additional testing can be done to evaluate your intellectual capabilities and aptitudes. The question may be whether you can return to your previous job position, another one similar to it, or if an entirely different position should be considered. The multidisciplinary pain-management center would be utilized for that purpose. Psychological testing results can be done for vocational counseling. A vocational counselor may already be involved in your management. If one has not been assigned, agencies are available that provide those services.

Job Placement

The success of your rehabilitation and acclimation to chronic pain is often based on job placement. First, an assessment of your capacity to return to your previous job is undertaken. As noted, the chronic pain patient is not likely to perform at the same functional level. Here, the vocational counselor plays a critical role by acting as a liaison to assess the workplace. Some modification of your job description may suffice for your return. Allowances for frequent rest periods, less time performing any given activity, changes in the number of working hours, or adjustments of the amount of weight lifted or carried may be possible. Often, employers will make those accommodations.

If your disability is greater, you might require some physical changes of the work environment or devices that will assist you. The Americans with Disabilities Act mandates accommodations within the work environment. Additions may be needed, where feasible. These include ramps, handrails, and changes to facilitate accessibility. You may need adaptive devices that would be used for fine manipulation or bracing. The vocational counselor would see to it that those devices are obtained and can be used at work. An assistant might be provided for some activities, if it is necessary.

The employer may not be able to institute these changes or the work environment may be unsuitable to accept these accommodations. Placement in a similar job would be considered. Applications and job interviews would be arranged by the counselor and you would receive instruction for the application process. In order to do this, some background knowledge of your previous work is necessary. For the most part, no additional skills or knowledge would be necessary.

If none of these options is available, another job position is considered. To do that, an evaluation of your educational background, aptitudes, preferences, and technical or professional training will give a clearer picture of your potentials. The multidisciplinary pain center is an ideal place to conduct this search. One may not be available, and referral would be made to a private clinician. The vocational counselor would be responsible for arranging the evaluation with a psychologist and social services for intelligence and aptitude testing. Based on results of those evaluations, a search for a vocation within your interests and capabilities could be directed. If necessary, vocational training would be given.

Analgesic Medication

Analgesic medication may never be completely discontinued. Some pain disorders, particularly complex regional pain syndromes, may require a maintenance prescription in combination with the other methods that have been discussed. I will not undertake a discussion of the medications that are prescribed, except to say that some of these are nonnarcotic medications such as nonsteroidal anti-inflammatories, and others are narcotics. The latter are referred to as opioids. Dependency on these medications has always been a concern of the medical profession. If used properly for severe chronic pain syndromes, though, they are appropriate. Some studies have shown that patients who warrant those prescriptions are capable of discontinuing the opioid when the pain syndrome has ceased.

If possible, reliance on pain medication is minimized. Certainly, there are going to be times when such medication is needed. After periods of increased activity or at the end of the day before retiring for sleep, over-the-counter or prescribed medication might need to be taken.

Less Conventional Treatments

The purpose of pain rehabilitation is to rely on means of management other than pain medication, such as attitudinal modification, relaxation, activity, and psychosocial support whenever possible. Less conventional forms of treatment can be continued. Acupuncture, for example, may not cure the problem or completely relieve the pain, but it may lessen the symptoms. Some clinical studies suggest that it can cause the release of endogenous analgesics similar to the release during exercise. Beware of people who promote themselves with unconventional methods of treatment that have not been shown to be of clinical value. They may attempt to take advantage of your defensive situation. For that reason, you should maintain an ongoing relationship with your physician to discuss these avenues of treatment. The chronic pain patient should be able to achieve an independent lifestyle, but periodic monitoring by your doctor is as necessary as it is for any other chronic illness.

SUGGESTED READINGS

Delisa, J.A. *Rehabilitation and Medicine, Principals and Practice,* 3d ed. Philadelphia: Lippincott-Raven Publishers, 1998.

Loeser, J.D., Bonica J.J. *Bonica's Management of Pain.* Philadelphia: Lippincott Williams & Wilkins, 2001.

Main, C.J., Spanswick, C.C. *Pain Management: An Interdisciplinary Approach.* Edinburgh, New York: Churchill Livingstone, 2000.

Simon, W.A., Ehrlich, G.E. *Medicolegal Consequences of Trauma.* New York: Marcel Dekker, 1993.

HELPFUL WEB SITES

American Academy of Pain Management
http://www.aapainmanage.org/

Chronic Pain Clearinghouse
http://www.myspirit2.homestead.com/home.html

Chronic Pain Management; The Pain Web
http://www.thepainweb.com/doclib/topics/000006.htm

Chronic Pain Solutions
http://www.chronicpainsolutions.com/recoreading.htm

Our Chronic Pain Mission; American Pain Foundation
http://www.cpmission.com/main/

Practice Guidelines for Chronic Pain Management; American Society of Anesthesiologists
http://www.asahq.org/practice/chronic_pain/chronic_pain.html

Treatment of Nonmalignant Chronic Pain; American Family Physician, 3/1/2000
http://www.aafp.org/afp/20000301/1331.html

Conclusion

In the "Tale of the Studious Locust," a chapter in the irreverent retelling by the Anglo-Indian author, Aubrey Menen, of the Hindu holy book, the *Ramayana,* the locust discovers that if one studies history one can predict the future exactly—provided things don't turn out differently. To some degree, that applies to medical prognosis. It's not an exact science, but one based on probabilities. Given the patient's complaints and their context, the physician can apply the knowledge and the vast experience communicated in textbooks and medical journals to come up with a plausible look into the future. But nature may contrive to vary that outlook slightly, as there are always situations that do not conform to the likeliest courses.

You have come this far, either by reading the whole book or by skipping around to find chapters that address your particular questions. You have learned that acute pain after an injury can lead to prolonged pain for a variety of reasons. Also, you have become aware that this chronic post-traumatic pain may lead to physical and emotional problems, apart from your original injury.

While physicians often have difficulty establishing the exact cause of your pain, some treatments may work for you and others may not, whether part of traditional medical care or part of alternative methods of care. Your concern about the future is legitimate, but no one can tell you precisely what will occur.

These variations in the results of treatment to individual patients are what color so-called "risk assessments." You always read in the daily newspapers that published medical studies have established that the risk of this and that happening is estimated at some percentage of likelihood. Yet all of us tend to act as if these assessments do not pertain to us. For example, it is now well established that smoking causes cancer and that it may cause or aggravate other diseases, some potentially fatal. Yet a considerable proportion of the population still smoke cigarettes. People who fear to fly because of the perceived risk of an accident will, on a daily basis, drive their SUVs on the crowded highways despite the greater risk, and they may drink one for the road despite the appalling rate of alcohol-related accidents and deaths.

The same principle applies to your medical status. The likelihood of recovery from even the most painful injuries is great, while the possibility of a drug reaction during treatment is minimal. Yet some people don't recover and do develop drug reactions. To maximize your chances of recovery and to minimize the possibility of reaction to strong analgesic or anti-inflammatory drugs, you must start by being honest and open with your physicians and by following sensible recommendations.

Moderate exercising is always good for you and should be instituted after the healing of your acute injuries, not just given lip service. Stopping smoking is an important aspect of your overall attempt to "get better." Your physician needs to know what else you are taking into your body besides prescribed medications. Herbals are drugs, even if available over the counter or in nutrition stores, and can influence your response to other medicines. Gingko biloba, for example, inhibits blood clotting, and if aspirin or other nonsteroidal anti-inflammatory drugs are prescribed or if you are taking an anticoagulant medicine, serious bleeding can result. Receiving manipulative therapy without your treating physician's knowledge can potentially produce complications. And while alternative medicine often helps to relieve chronic post-traumatic pain, as previous chapters have shown, it should not become a substitute for appropriate medical care; it should act as a complement. Nor should your use of alternative treatment be kept from your physician (although estimates suggest that almost half of patients using alternative medicine don't inform their doctors!).

Adopt healthful habits. Wear seat belts. Eat intelligently; there are few harmful foods if they are eaten in moderation, but even eating healthful foods and following diets can cause harm if they are taken to the extreme. Be reasonable. Focus on the things that really matter and don't exaggerate risks.

Perhaps you should read John Allen Paulos's book *Innumeracy* to gain a perspective on which risks are real and which aren't (you rarely learn this from reading the scary stories in the newspapers or watching the sound bites on television). An important point to remember is that an association need not necessarily mean causation. Common events often occur together, and therefore a *causal* relationship, which may seem to be common sense, in reality is merely a *casual* relationship. Don't be one of the people who trumpets, "I am the evidence," that one event brought on the other. The overwhelming odds are that you aren't.

Certainly, the tragic events of September 11, 2001, have helped us all to gain a new perspective on life, to appreciate what we have, and to try to live each day with gratitude. Keep a realistic perspective; emphasize how much remains that makes us human and how little we have lost as a consequence of our individual injuries. Keeping an eye on the positive elements in our lives will help dispel pessimism and depression and help bring our pains to levels we can tolerate. Letting pain rule your life is definitely counterproductive.

This book has attempted to tell you a little bit more about yourself. It has helped explain the origins of post-traumatic pain, and has informed you about the various ways people around the world address their pain. Not all the remedies in this book have been medically or scientifically verified, even though many are supported by individual testimonials. However, the editors believe that it is important to tell you about the various means that others have used to gain relief from chronic pain while not necessarily advocating the curative value of all these approaches.

The best rule to follow might be to trust your health-care professional and your personal recuperative strength, to have hope, and to move forward with your productive life. Good luck!

George E. Ehrlich, M.D.

INDEX

About the Authors

EDITORS

William H. Simon, M.D., F.A.C.S., is a clinical associate professor of orthopedic surgery at the University of Pennsylvania School of Medicine.

George E. Ehrlich, M.D., F.A.C.P., M.A.C.R., is an adjunct professor of medicine at the University of Pennsylvania School of Medicine and an adjunct professor of medicine at New York University School of Medicine.

Arnold Sadwin, M.D., F.A.P.M., F.P.C.P., was an assistant clinical professor of psychiatry and neurology in the Department of Psychiatry at the University of Pennsylvania School of Medicine until he retired. He is clinical assistant professor in the Department of Family Practice at the University of Medicine & Dentistry of New Jersey.

CONTRIBUTORS

Arvind Chopra, M.D., is a consultant rheumatologist and honorary associate professor of medicine at the Center for Rheumatic Diseases, Bharatiya Vidyapeeth Hospital and Medical College in Pune, India.

Jennifer Chu, M.D., is an associate professor of physical medicine and rehabilitation at the University of Pennsylvania School of Medicine.

Jano Cohen is a bodywork expert, lecturer, and instructor.

Marian Garfinkel, Ed.D., is a faculty lecturer at the School of Nursing Education, MCP-Hahnemann University in Philadelphia, Pennsylvania, and is the director of the BKS Iyengar Yoga Studio of Philadelphia.

Sanjay Gupta, M.D., is the chief of the Pain Center at Albert Einstein Medical Center, Philadelphia, Pennsylvania.

Gloria Horwitz, M.S., is a psychologist and nutrition consultant.

Sharon L. Kolasinski, M.D., is an assistant professor of medicine and the chief of clinical service in the Division of Rheumatology at the University of Pennsylvania School of Medicine.

Elizabeth Michel, M.D., is a family practitioner.

Joseph C. Napoli, M.D., F.A.P.A., is an assistant clinical professor of phychiatry at the College of Physicians and Surgeons of Columbia University.

Andrew Newberg, M.D., is an assistant professor of radiology at the University of Pennsylvania School of Medicine.

Jayshree Patil, M.D., is an Ayurvedic physician and research associate at the Center for Rheumatic Diseases in Pune, India.

Bruce Pfleger, Ph.D., is a musculoskeletal epidemiology consultant at the chronic disease management section of The World Health Organization (WHO), Geneva, Switzerland.

Barry Snyder, M.D., F.A.C.S., is an associate faculty member at the University of Pennsylvania School of Medicine, Department of Orthopedic Surgery.